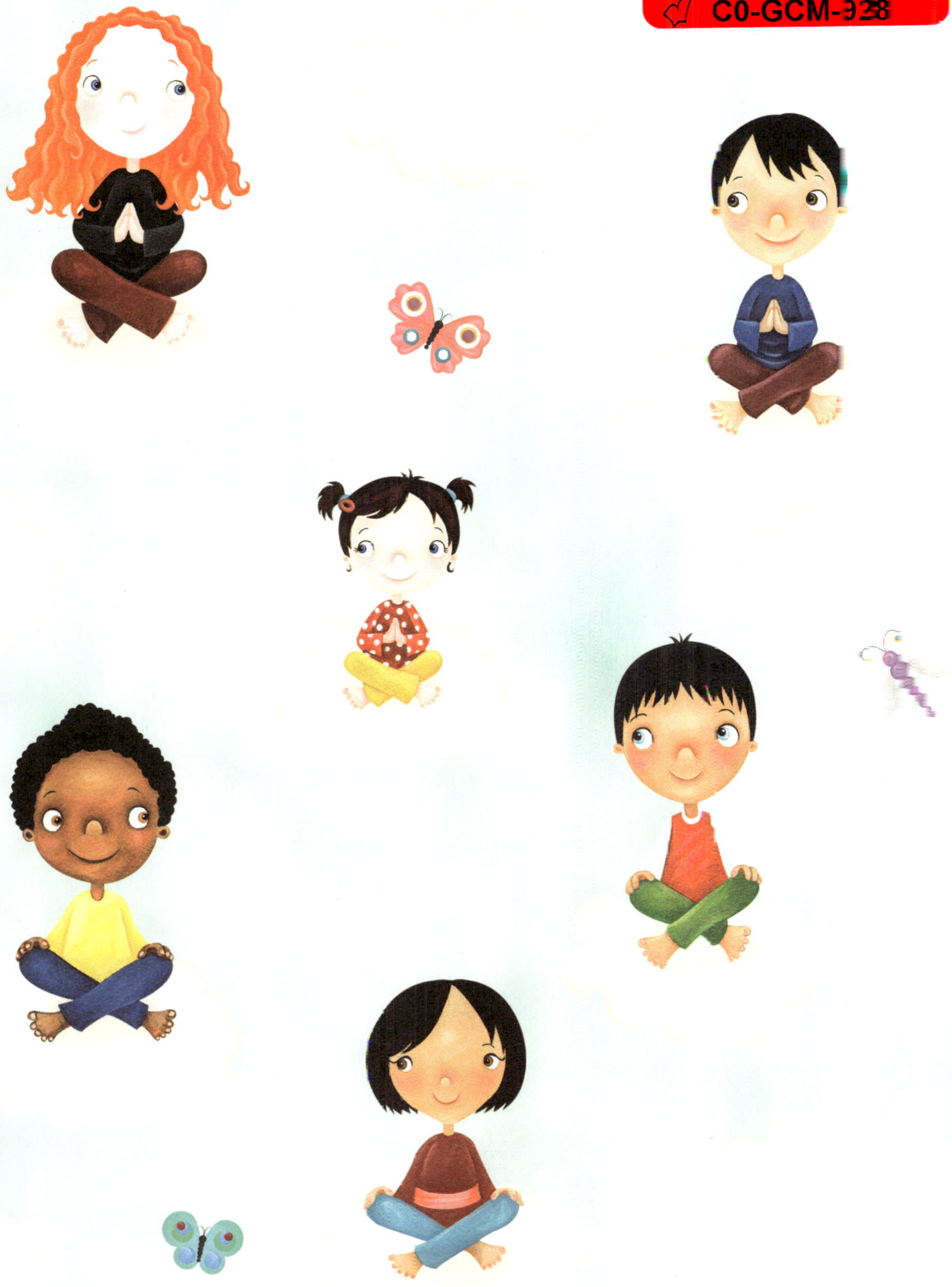

good night yoga

a pose-by-pose bedtime story

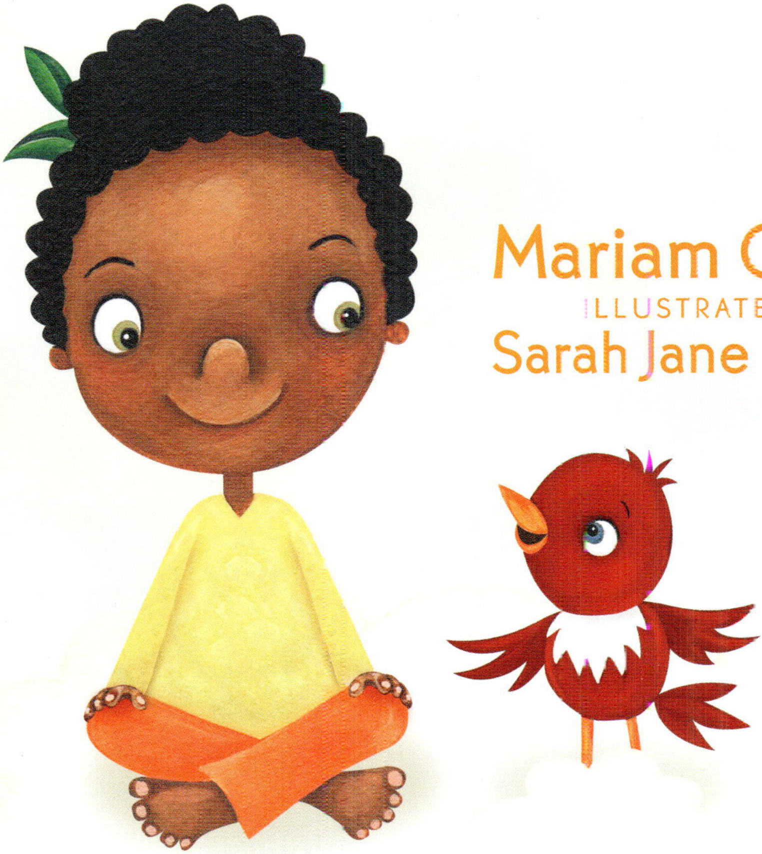

Mariam Gates
ILLUSTRATED BY
Sarah Jane Hinder

SOUNDS TRUE
BOULDER, COLORADO

Sounds True
Boulder, CO 80306

Published 2015

Book design by Beth Skelley
Printed in Korea

Library of Congress Cataloging-in-Publication Data
Gates, Mariam.
Good night yoga : a pose-by-pose bedtime story / Mariam Gates ;
illustrated by Sarah Jane Hinder.
pages cm
Audience: 3 & up
Audience: K to Grade 3
ISBN 978-1-62203-466-6—ISBN 978-1-62203-470-3 (Ebook)
1. Hatha yoga for children—Juvenile literature.
I. Hinder, Sarah Jane, illustrator. II. Title.
RJ133.7.G42 2015
613.7'046083—dc23
2014043295

ISBN 978-1-62203-466-6
Ebook ISBN 978-1-62203-470-3

10 9

For the three of you—Rolf, Jasmine, and Dylan.

MG

To Mike, my best friend and husband, for all your love
and support, and for the hot chocolates when I'm working.
For Dan, the best son ever! For my little inspirations:
Josh, Meg, Katie and Bridie, Isabel, Ava, Ellie and William.

SJH

The sun in the sky is going down

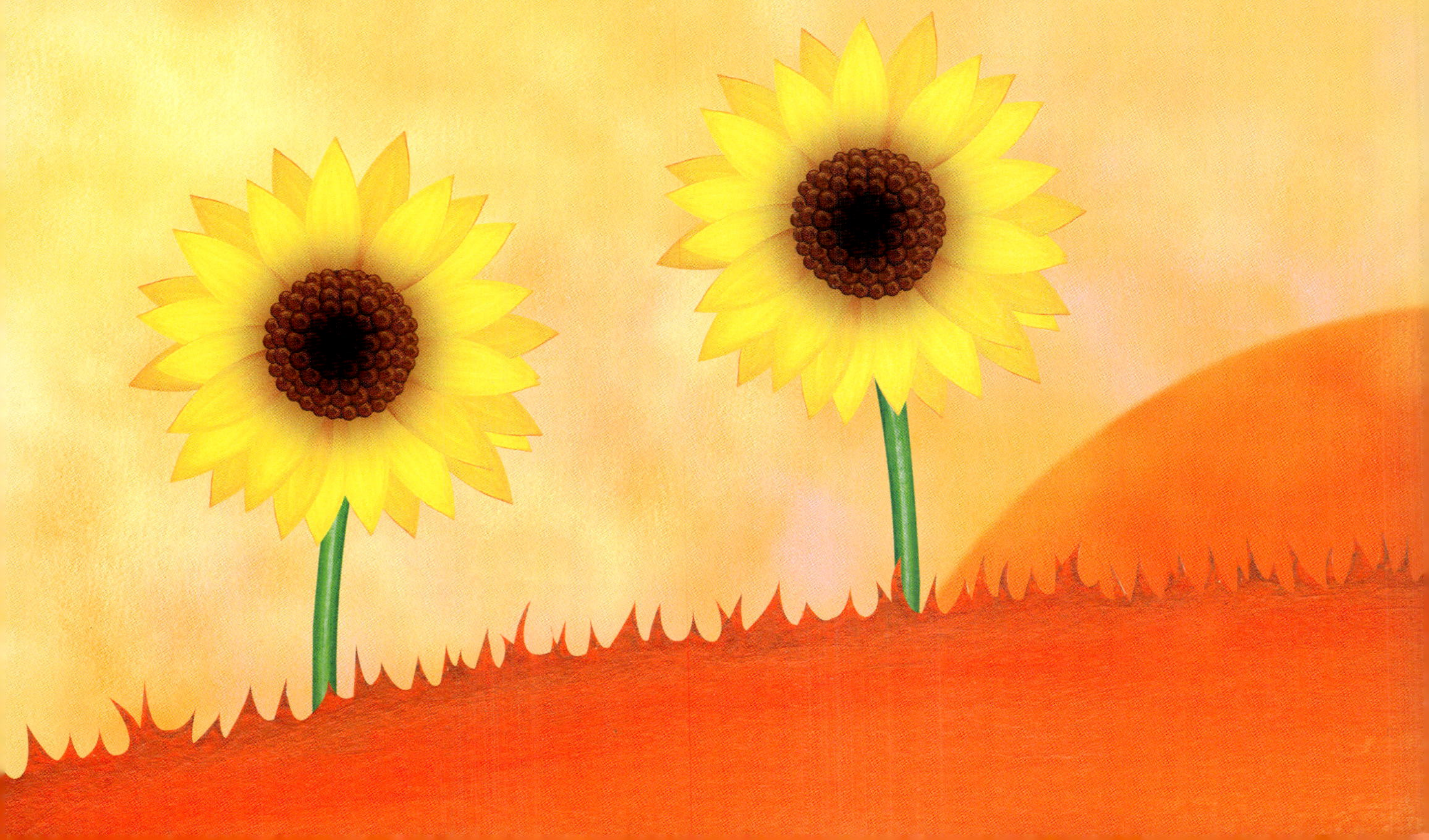

As I breathe in, as I breathe out,
my arms lift up to the sky
and then back down like sunrays.

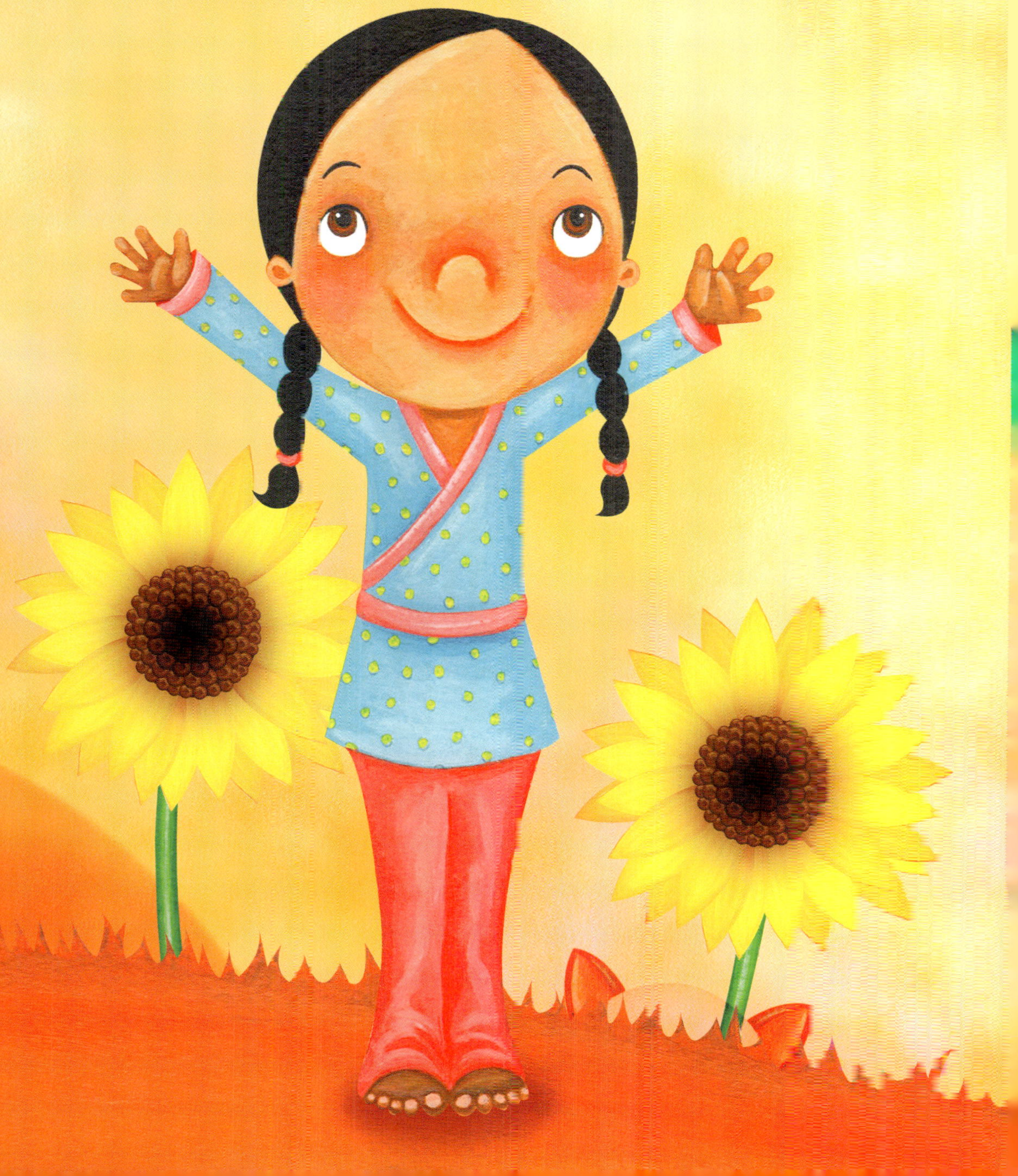

As I breathe in, I bend my knees
and scoop the clouds around me.
As I breathe out, I stand tall
and release the clouds over my head.

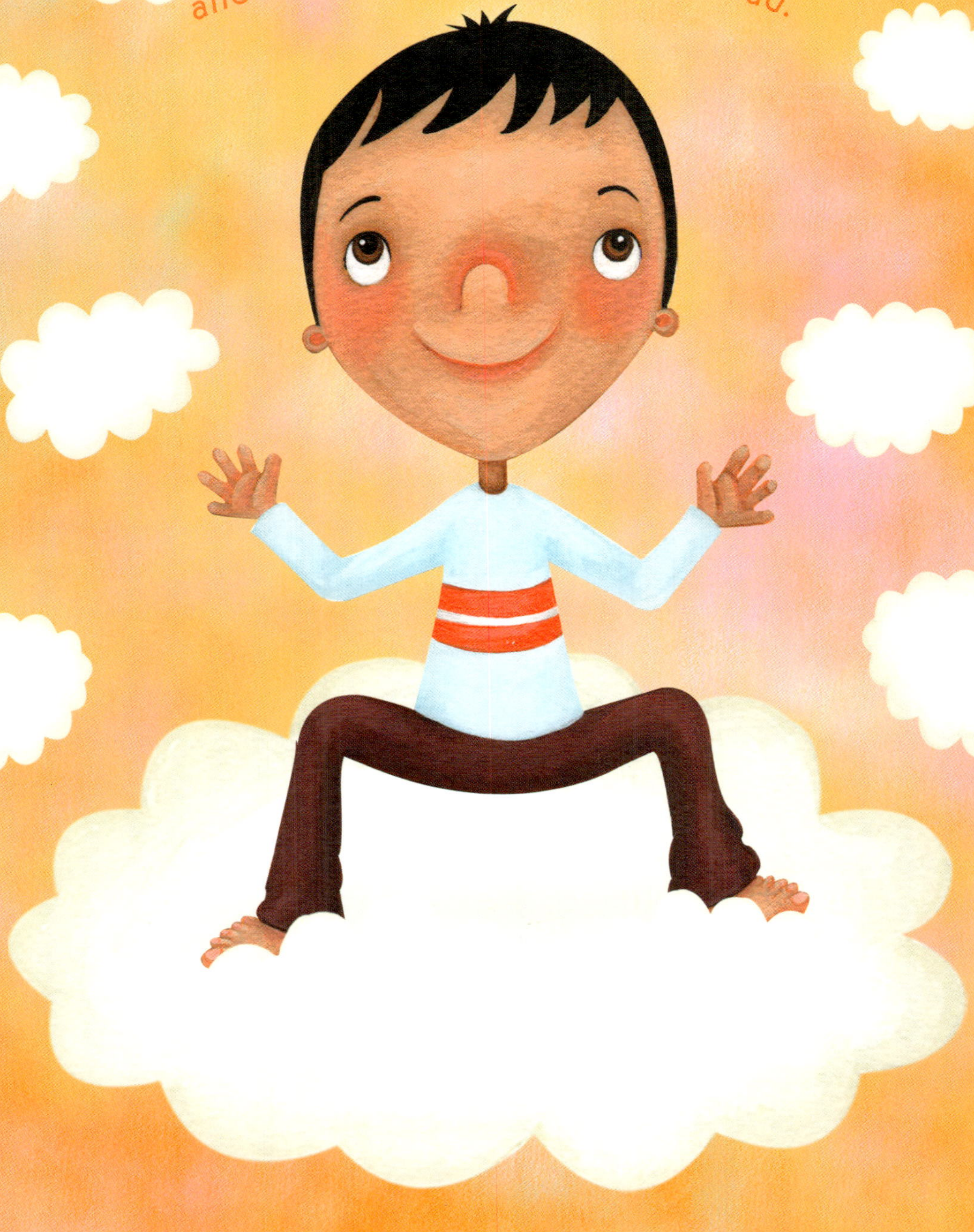

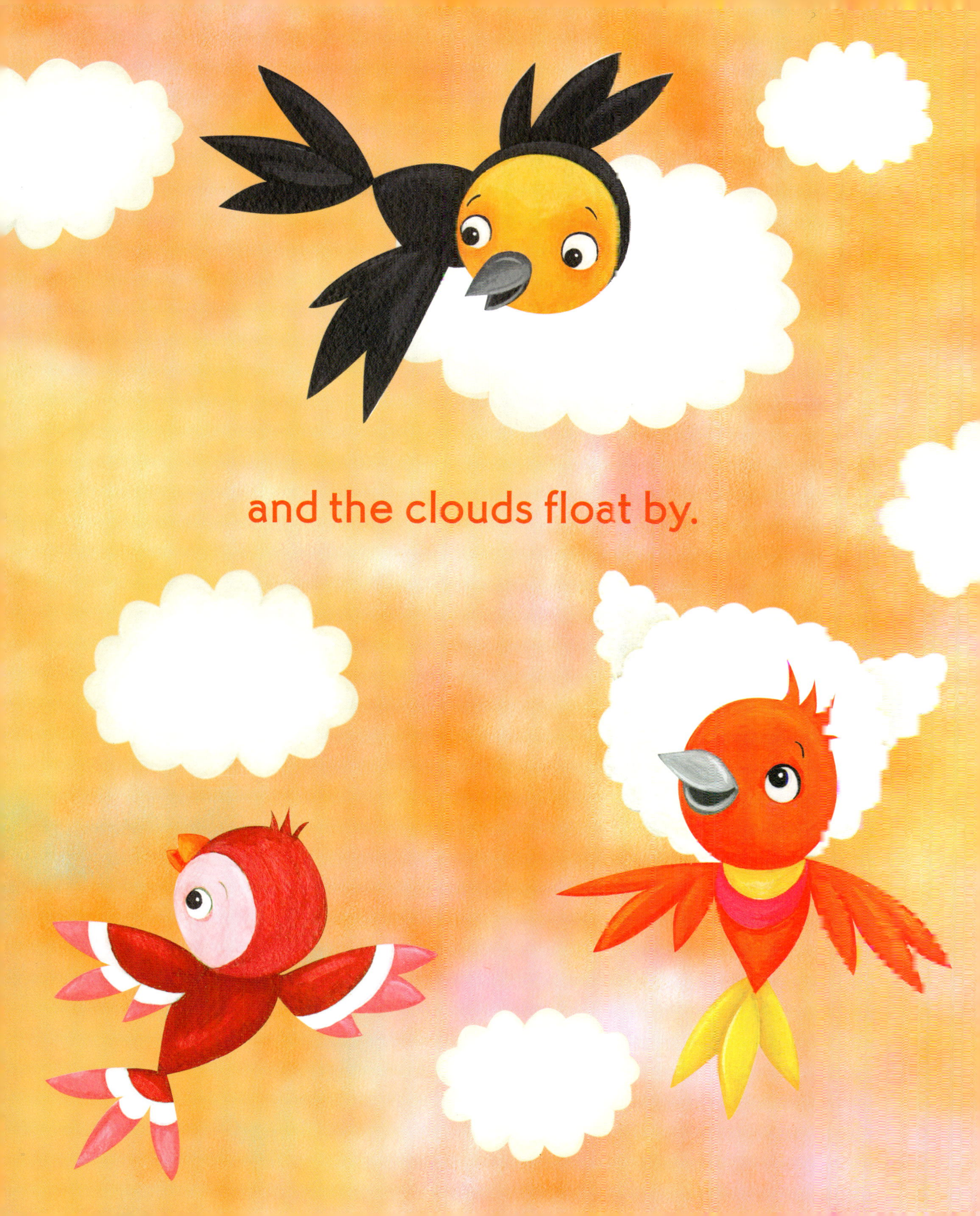

and the clouds float by.

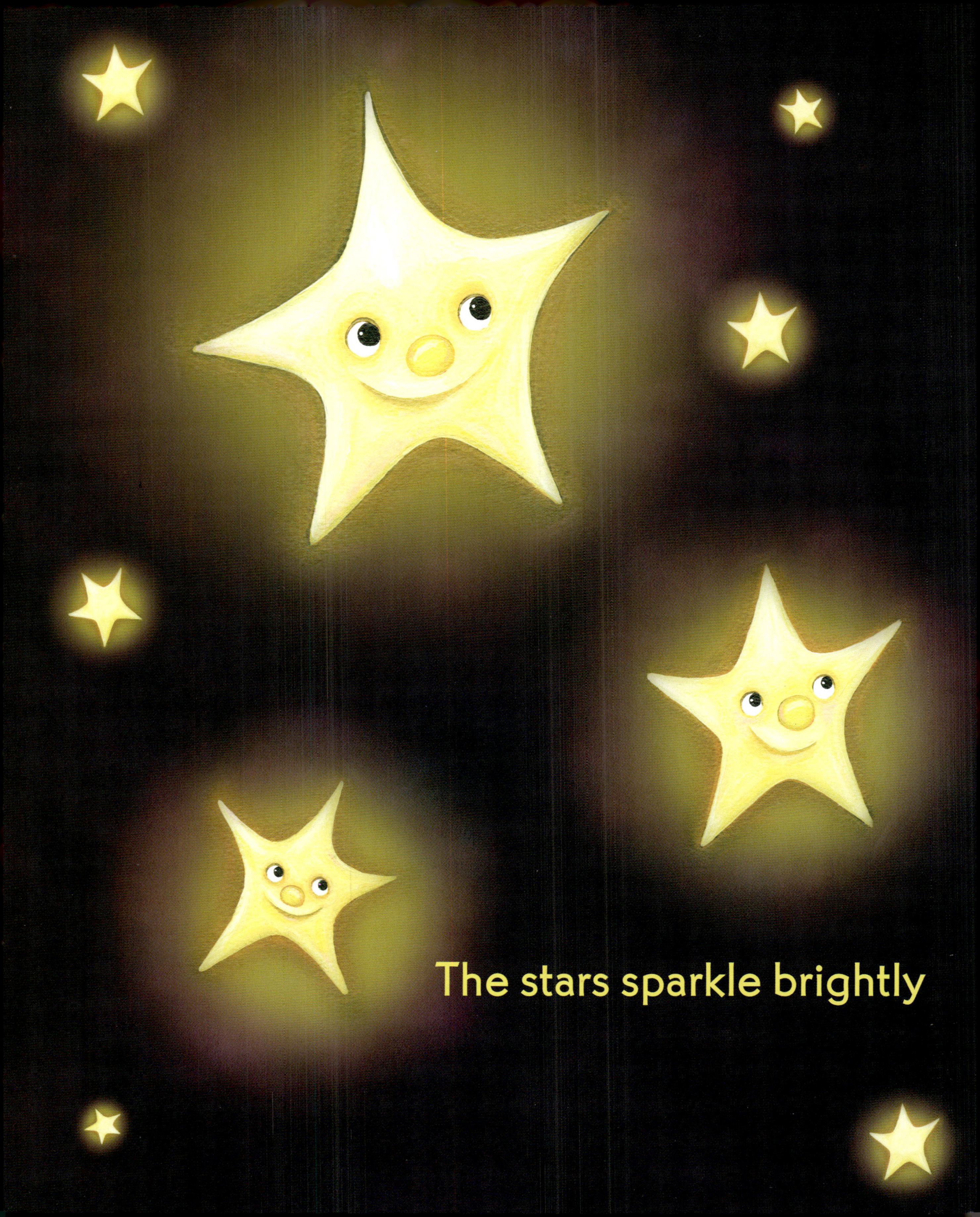

The stars sparkle brightly

As I breathe in, as I breathe out,
my arms reach out
wide toward the stars.

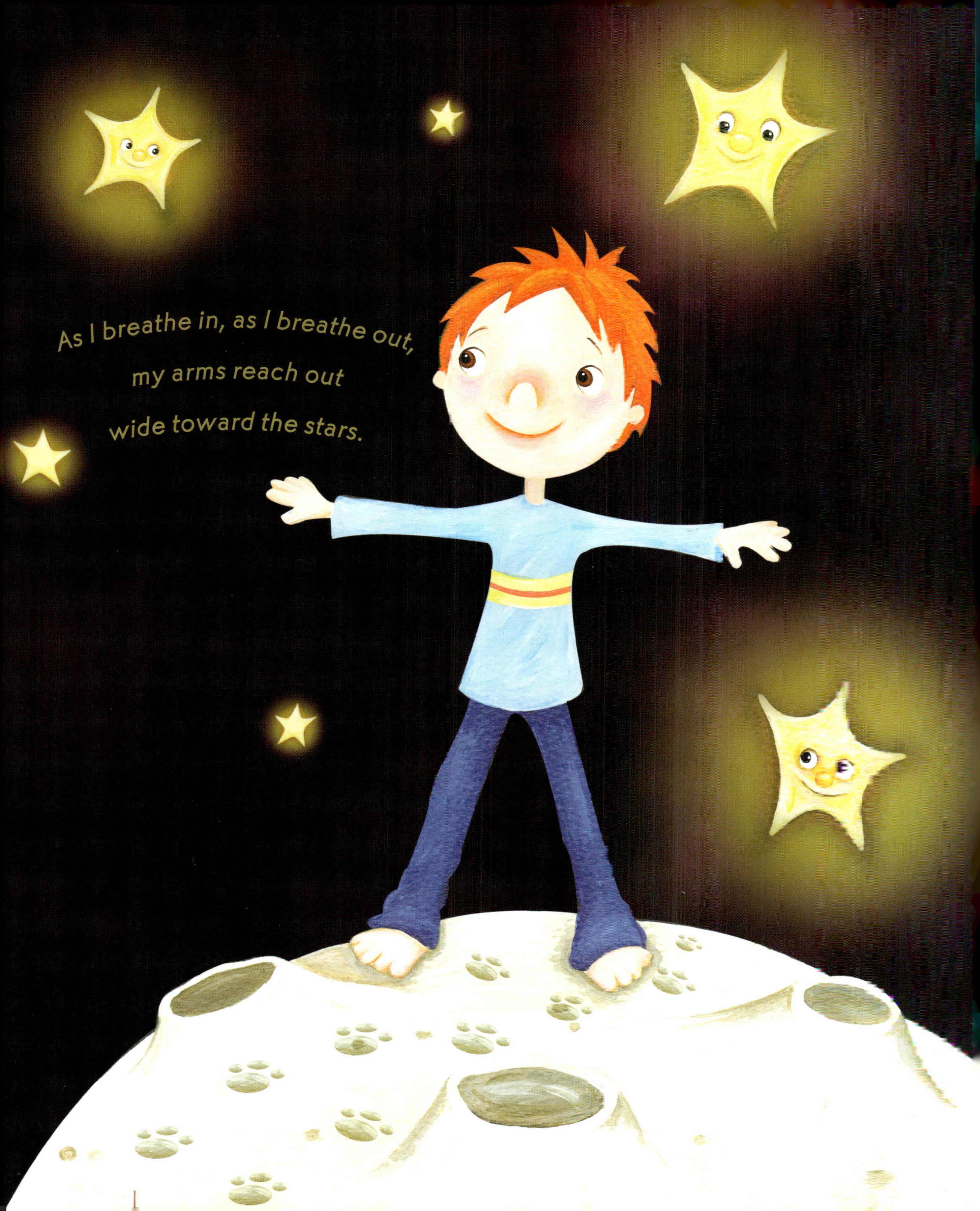

as the moon rises high.

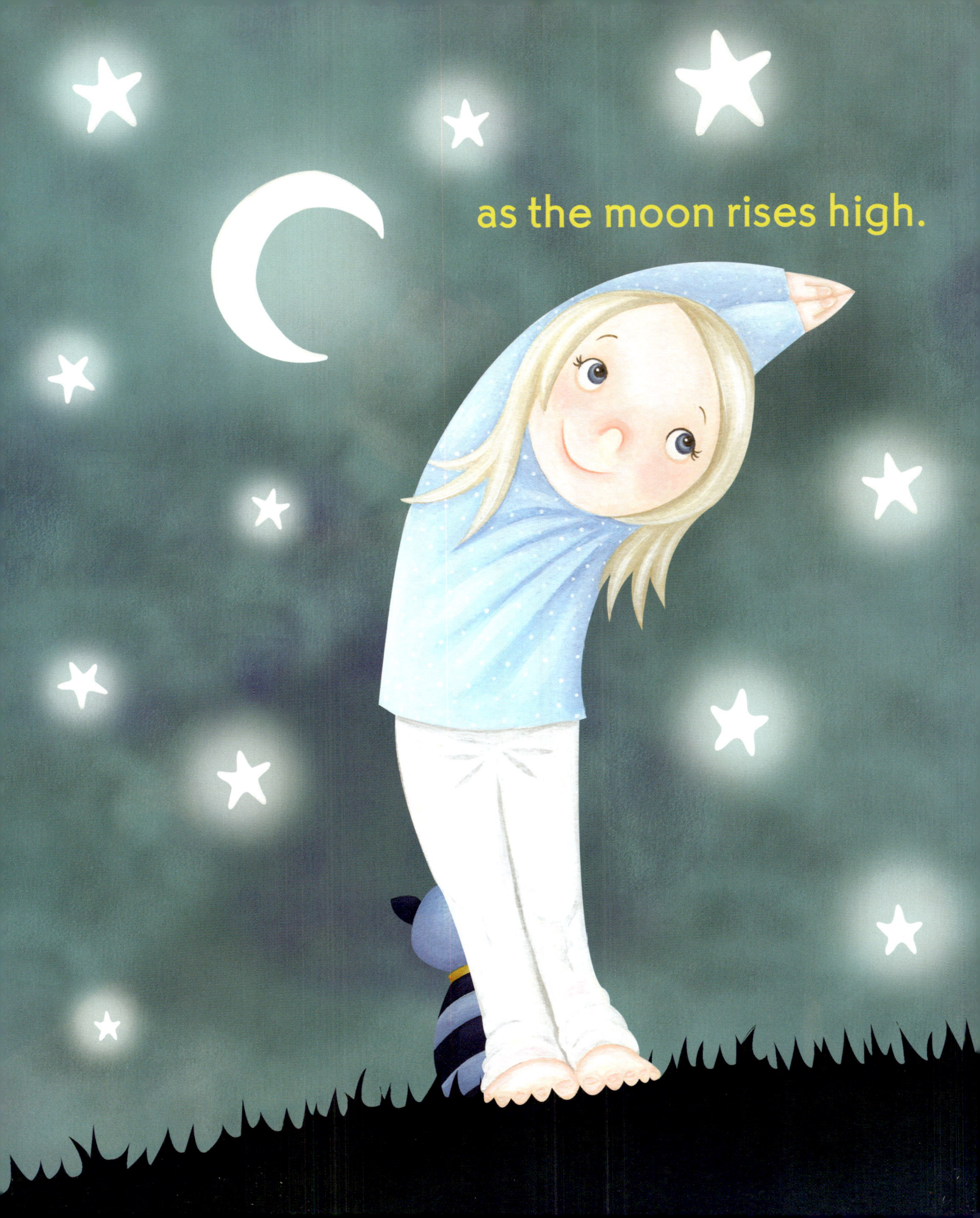

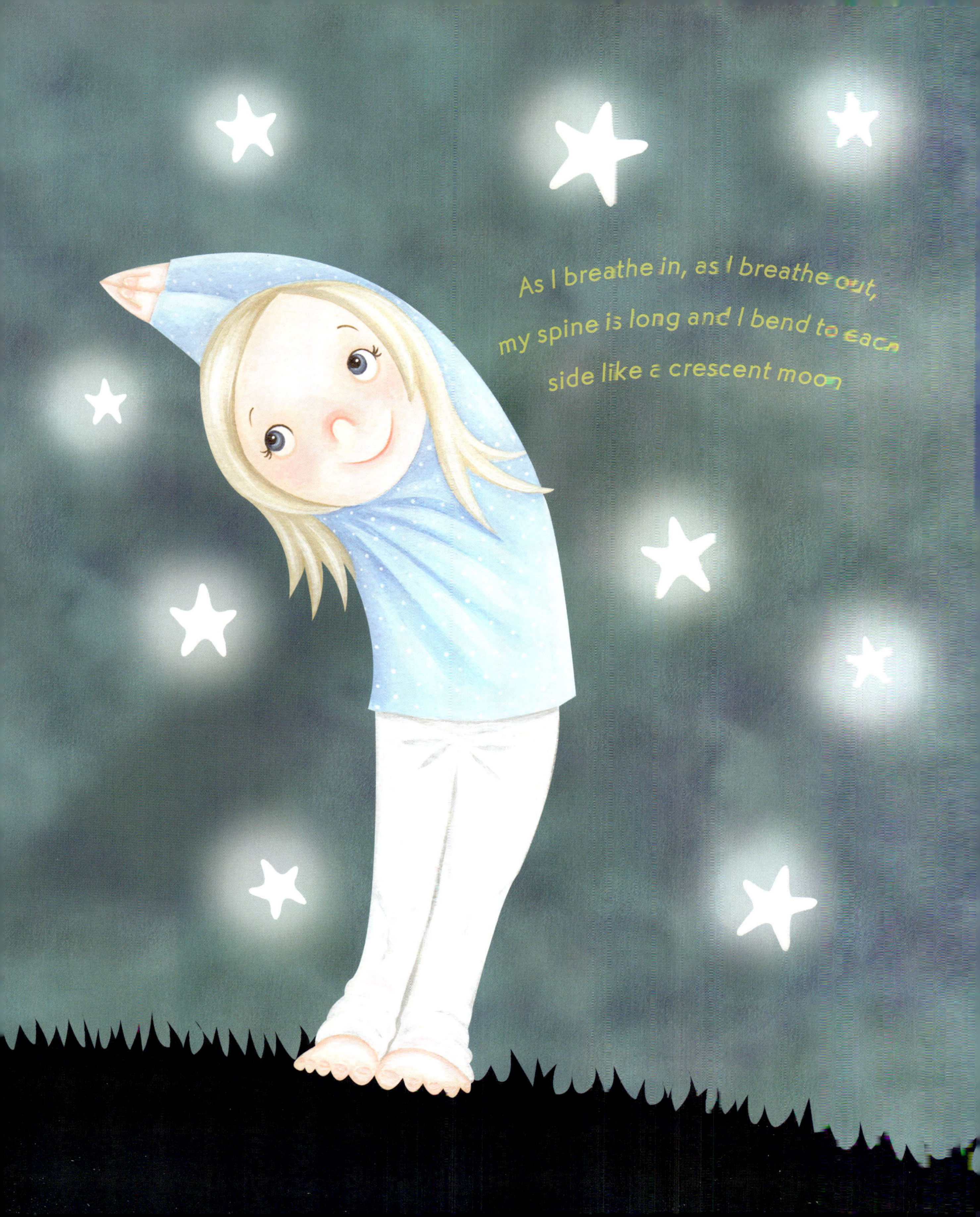

As I breathe in, as I breathe out,
my spine is long and I bend to each
side like a crescent moon

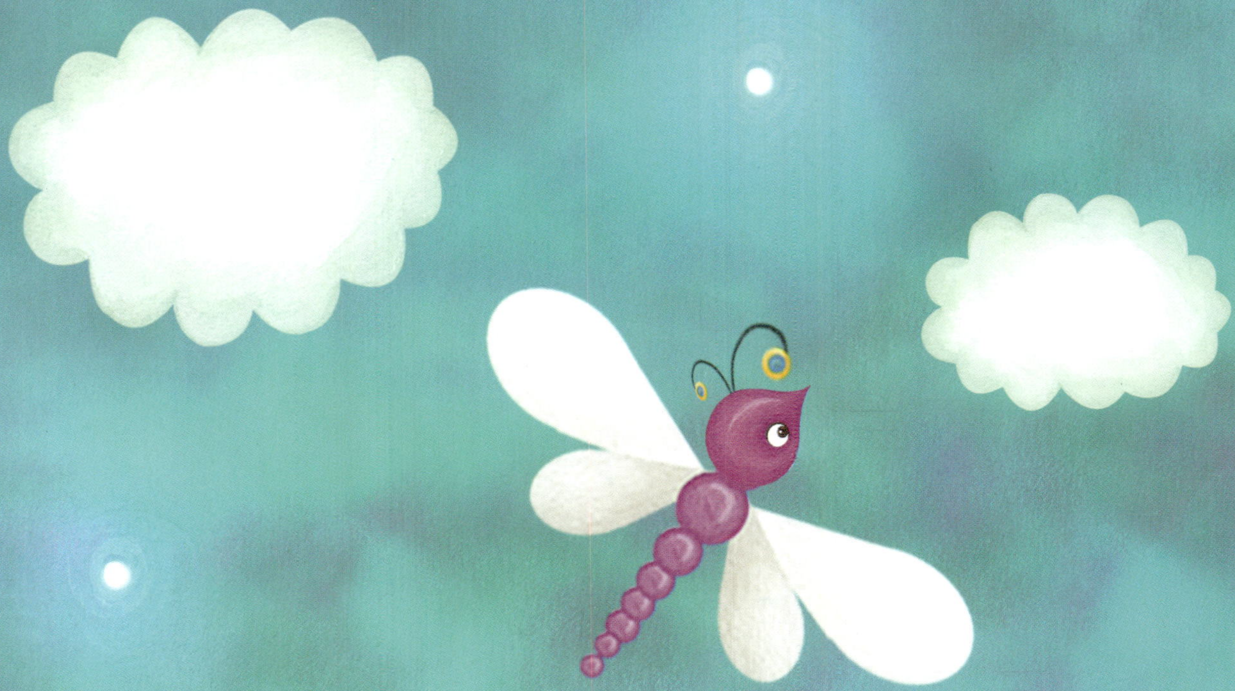

The birds are flying back now

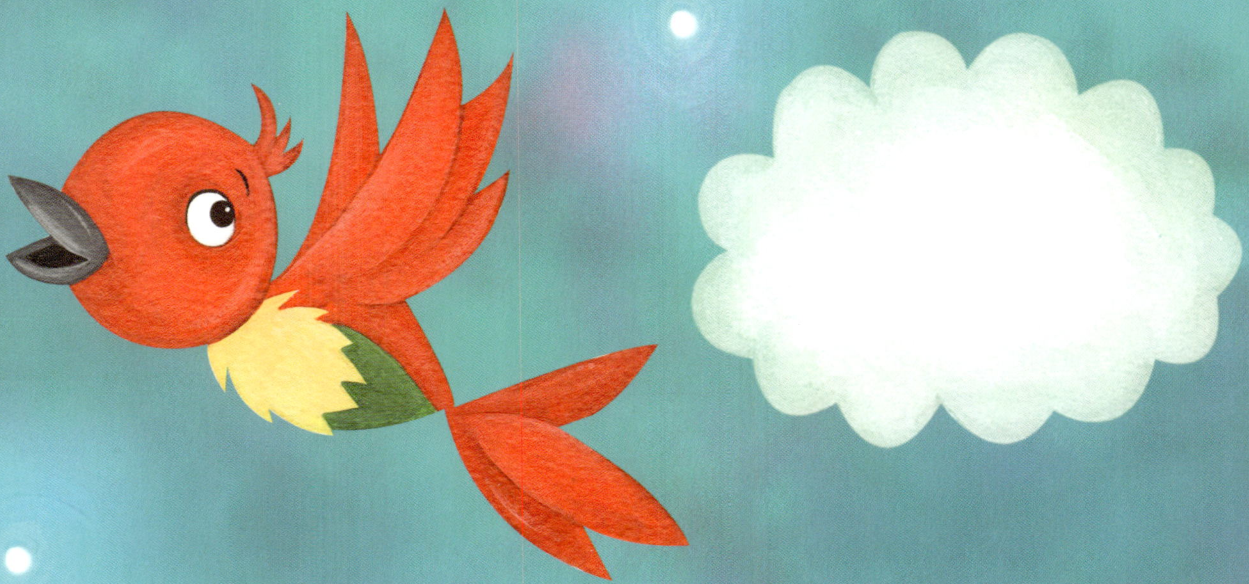

As I breathe in, as I breathe out,
I focus on one point
and use my arms to soar.

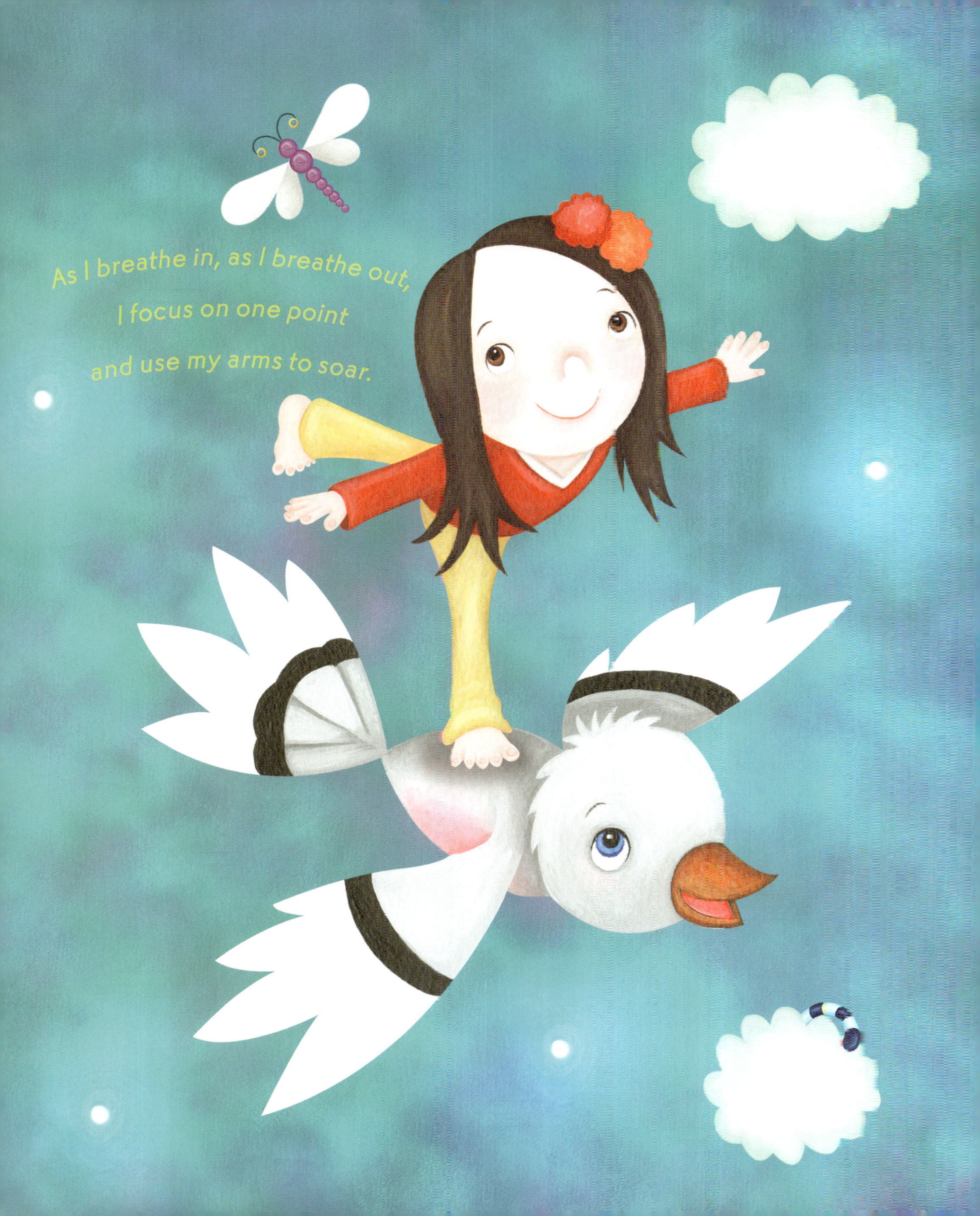

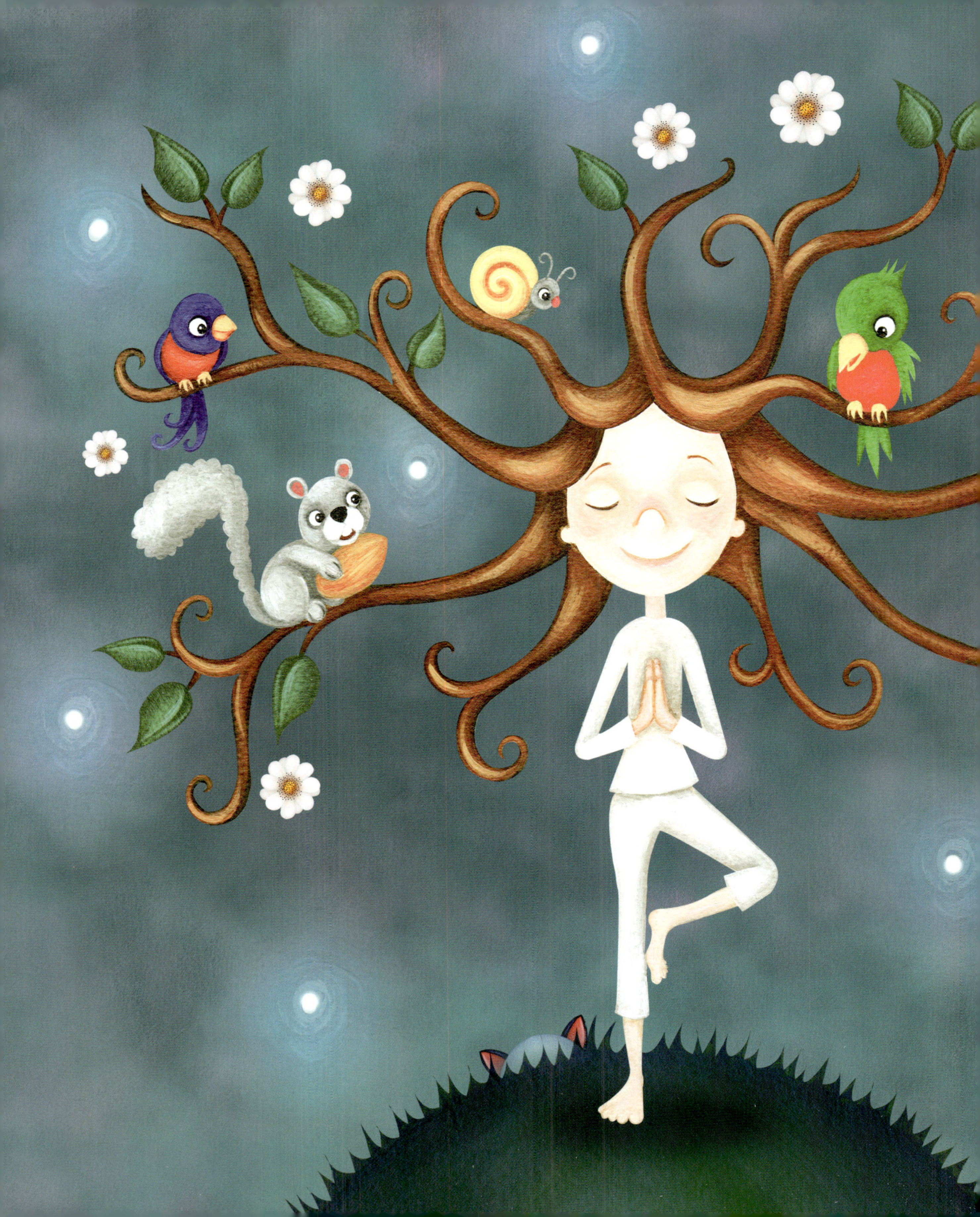

As I breathe in, as I breathe out,
my shoulders roll back,
my heart is open,
and I am solid like a tree.

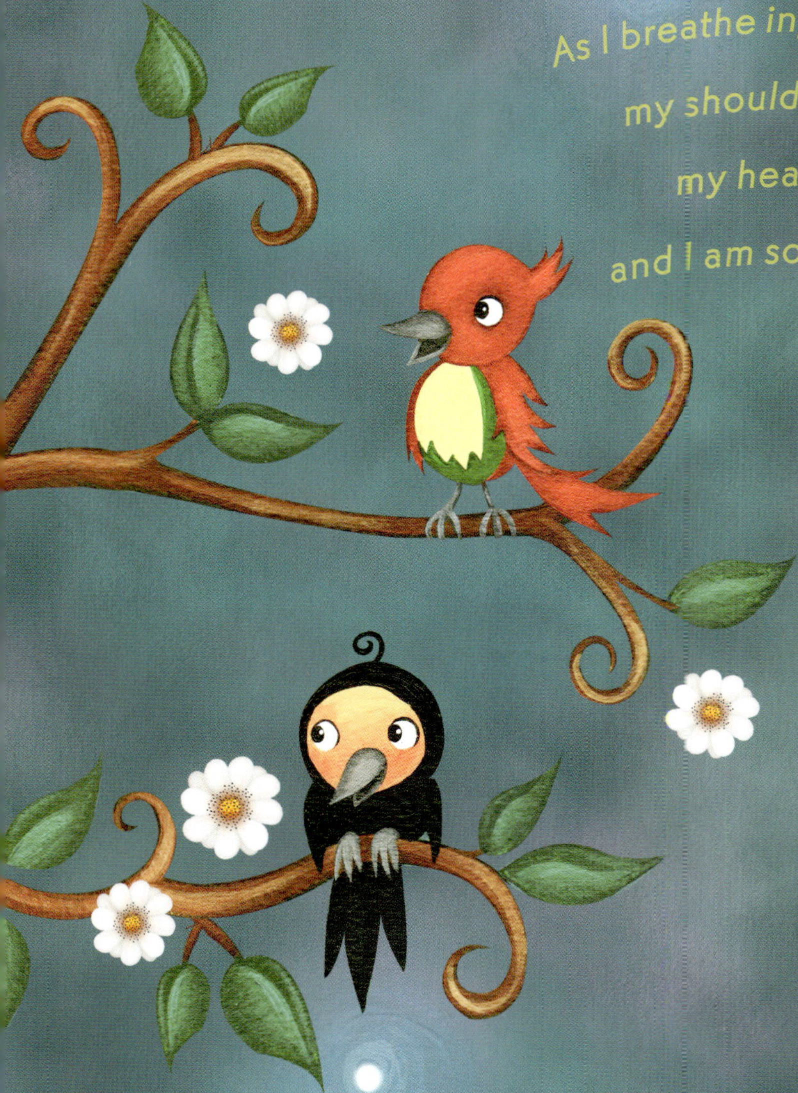

to their homes in the trees.

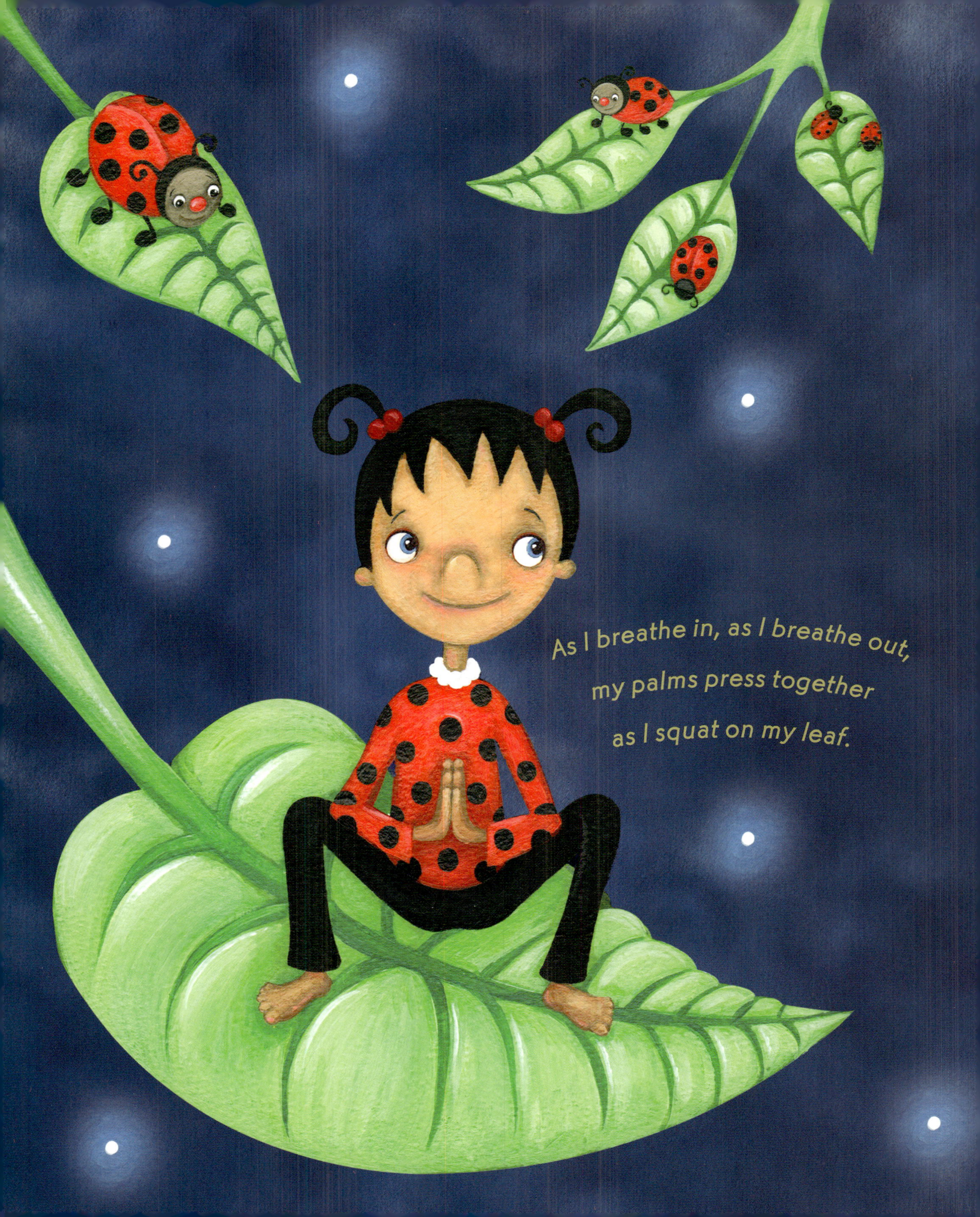

As I breathe in, as I breathe out,
my palms press together
as I squat on my leaf.

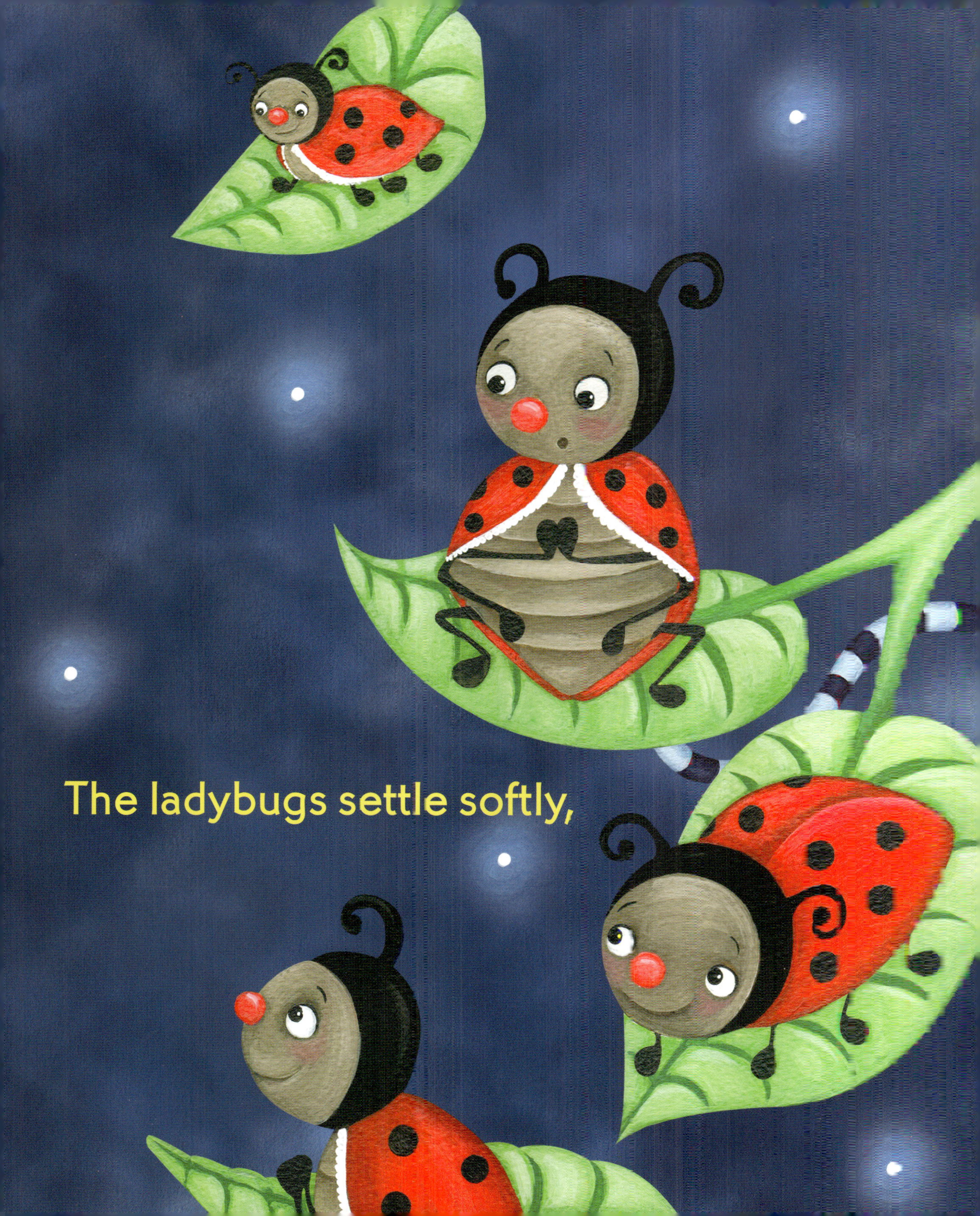

The ladybugs settle softly,

As I breathe in, as I breathe out,
my feet press together
and my knees spread out
like butterfly wings.

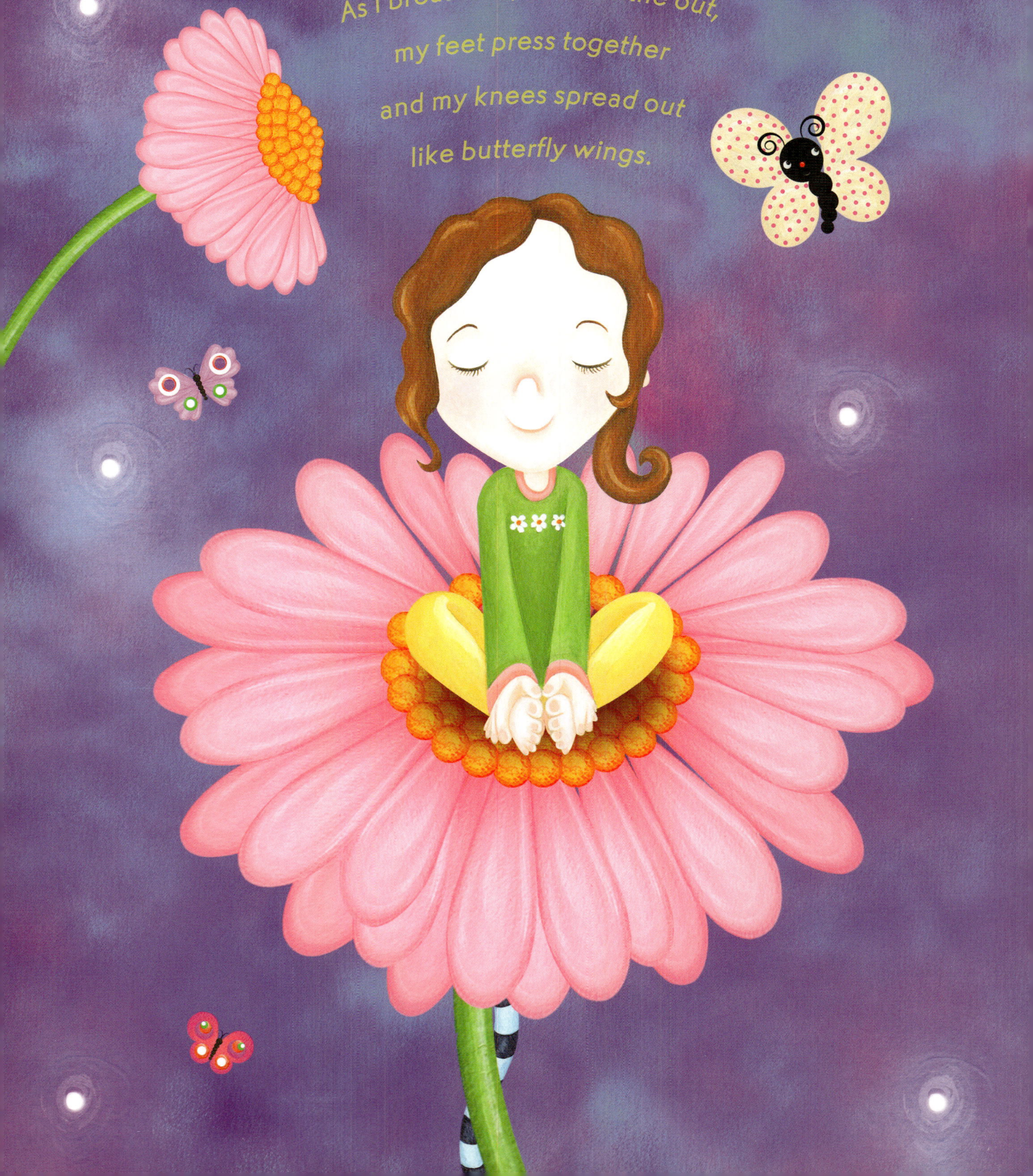

between the butterflies

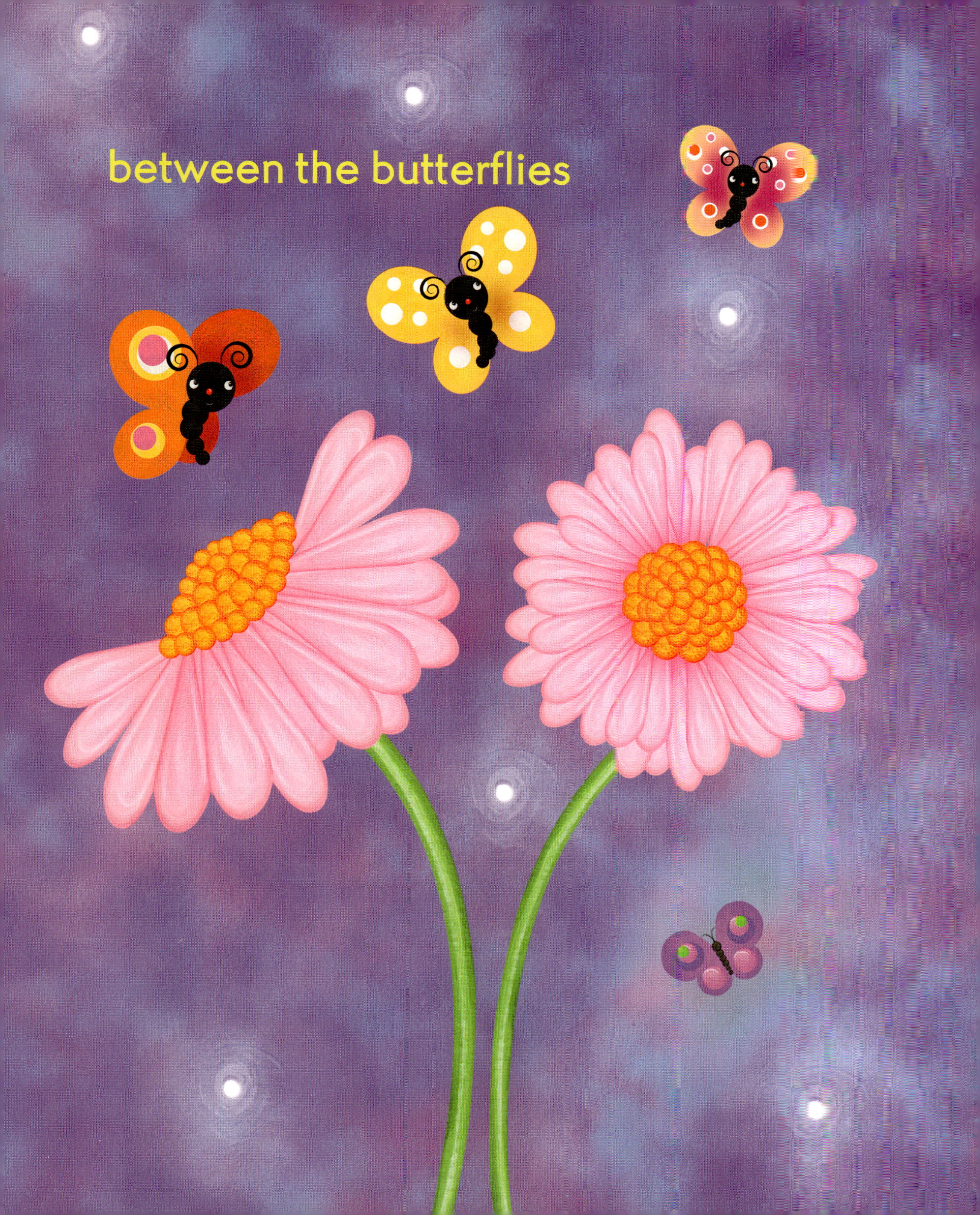

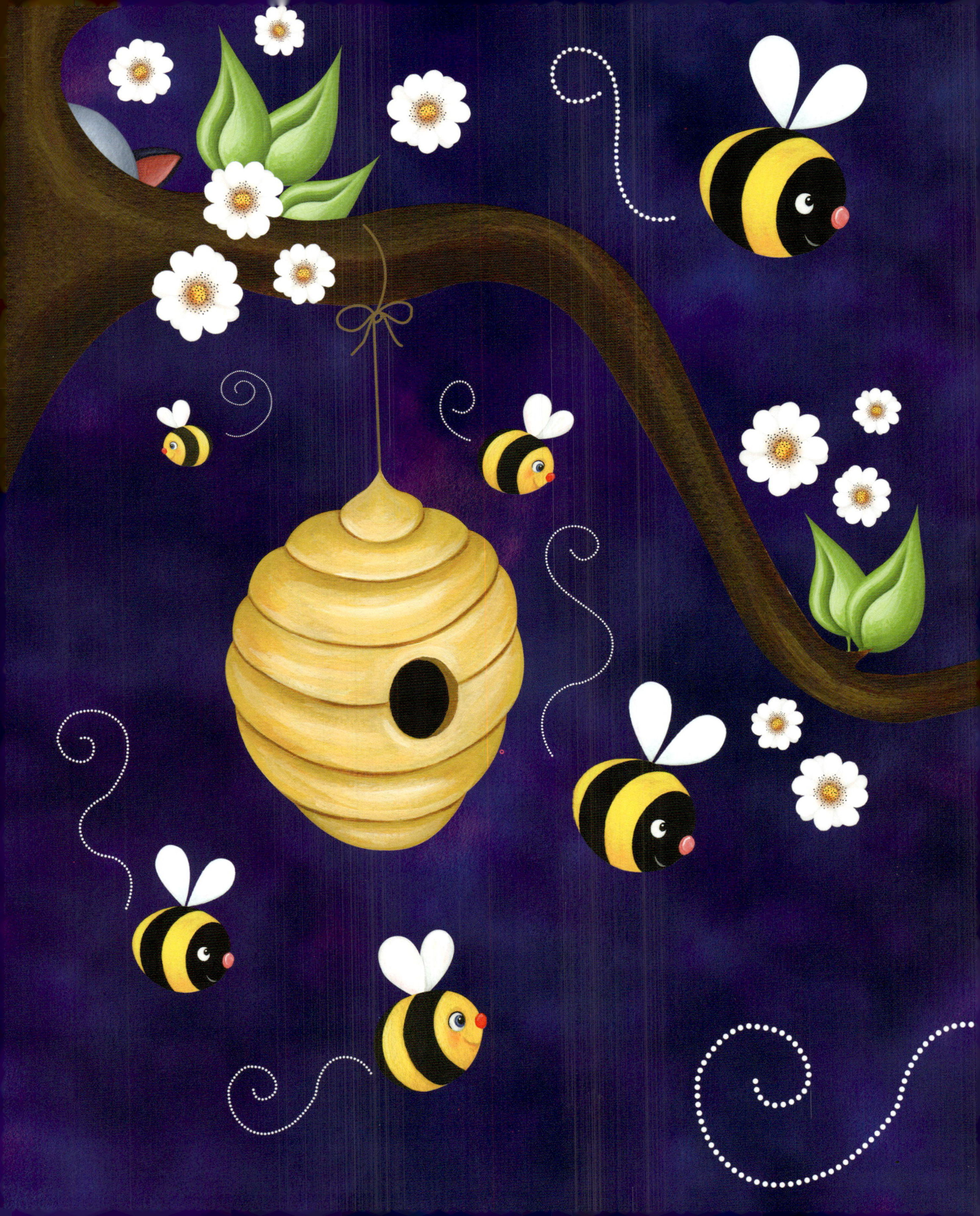

As I breathe in, I sit up tall
and reach my arms back like wings.
As I breathe out, I buzz
my head down to the ground.

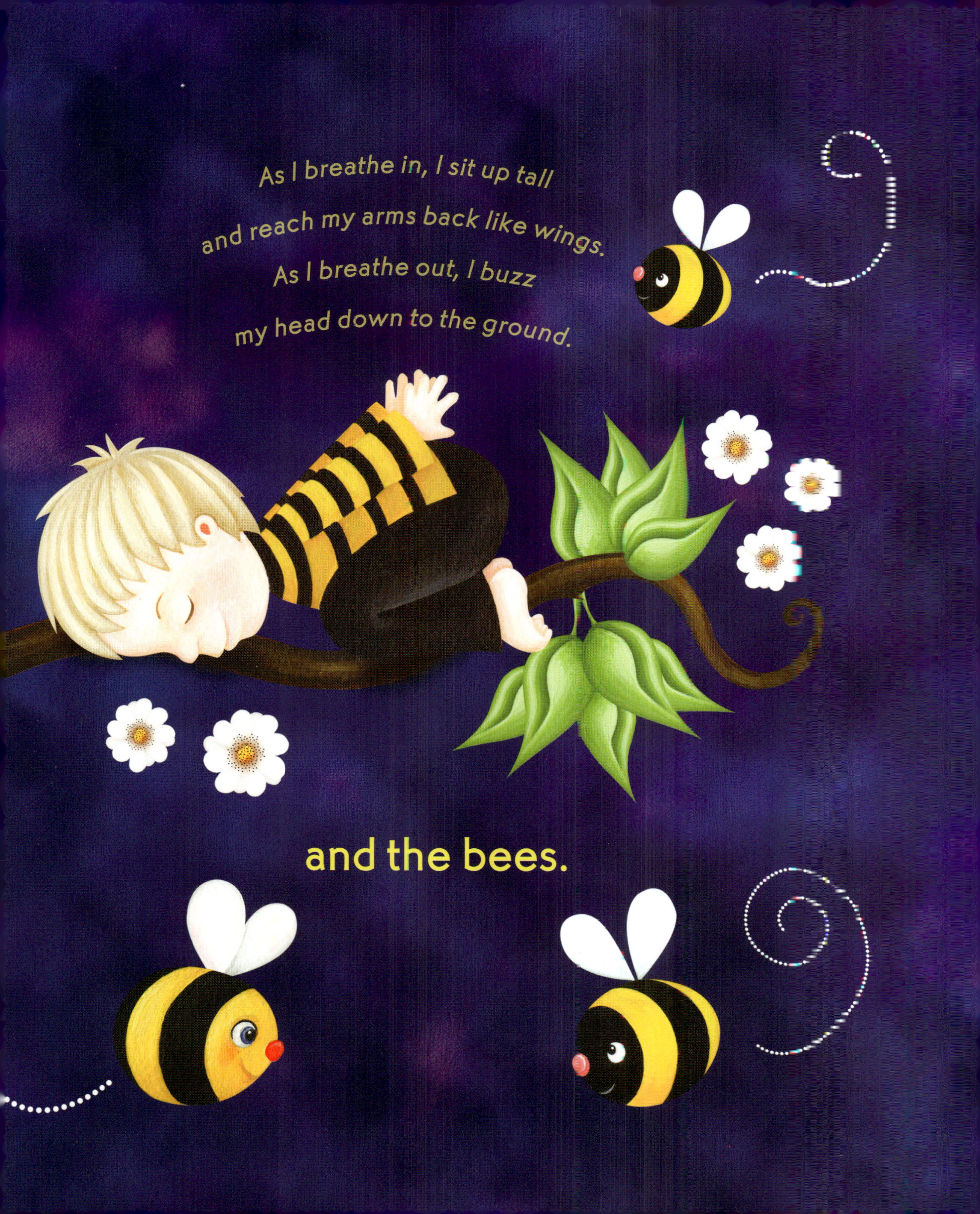

and the bees.

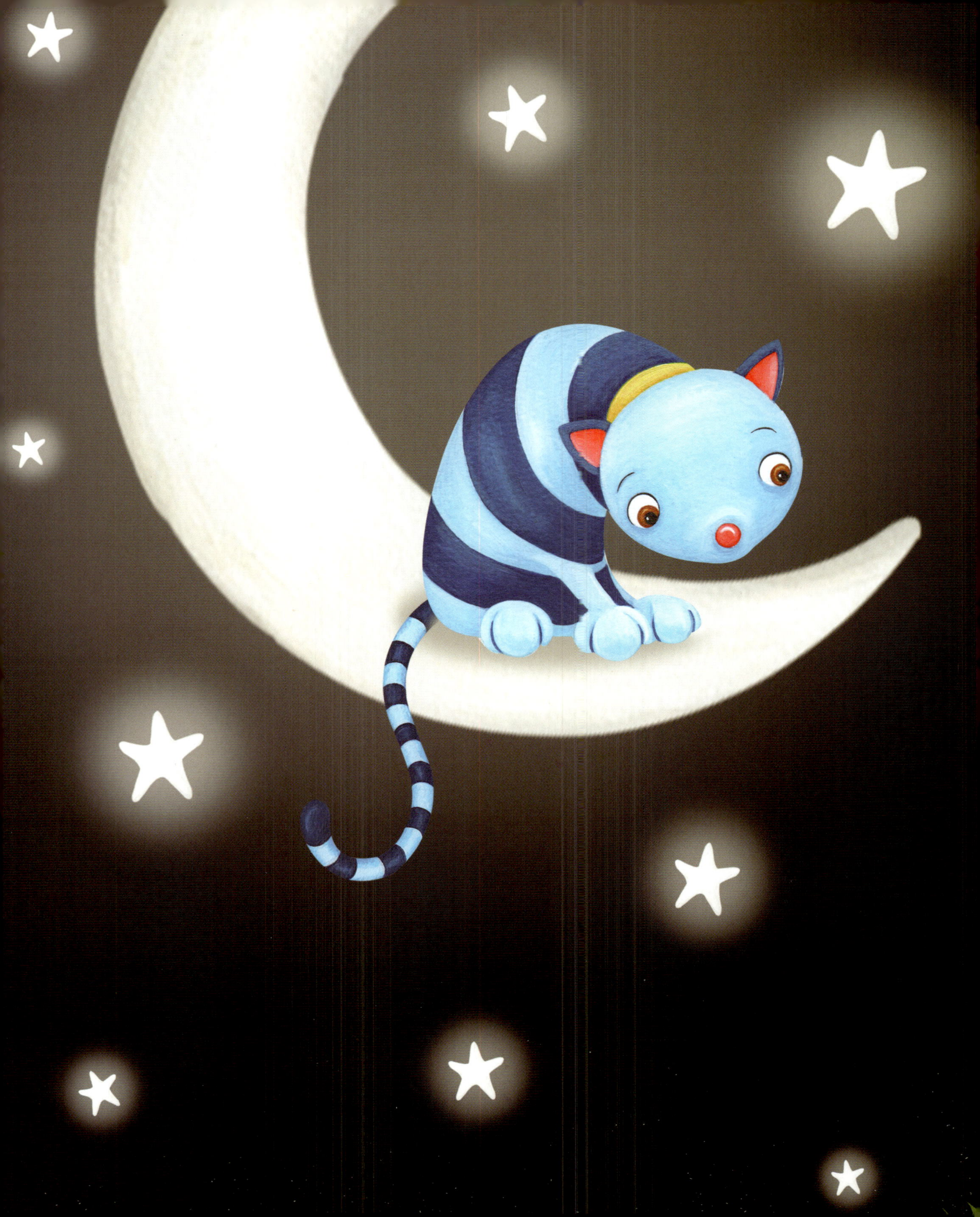

The little blue cat,
who lives in the moon,

As I breathe in, as I breathe out,
I arch my back like a cat.

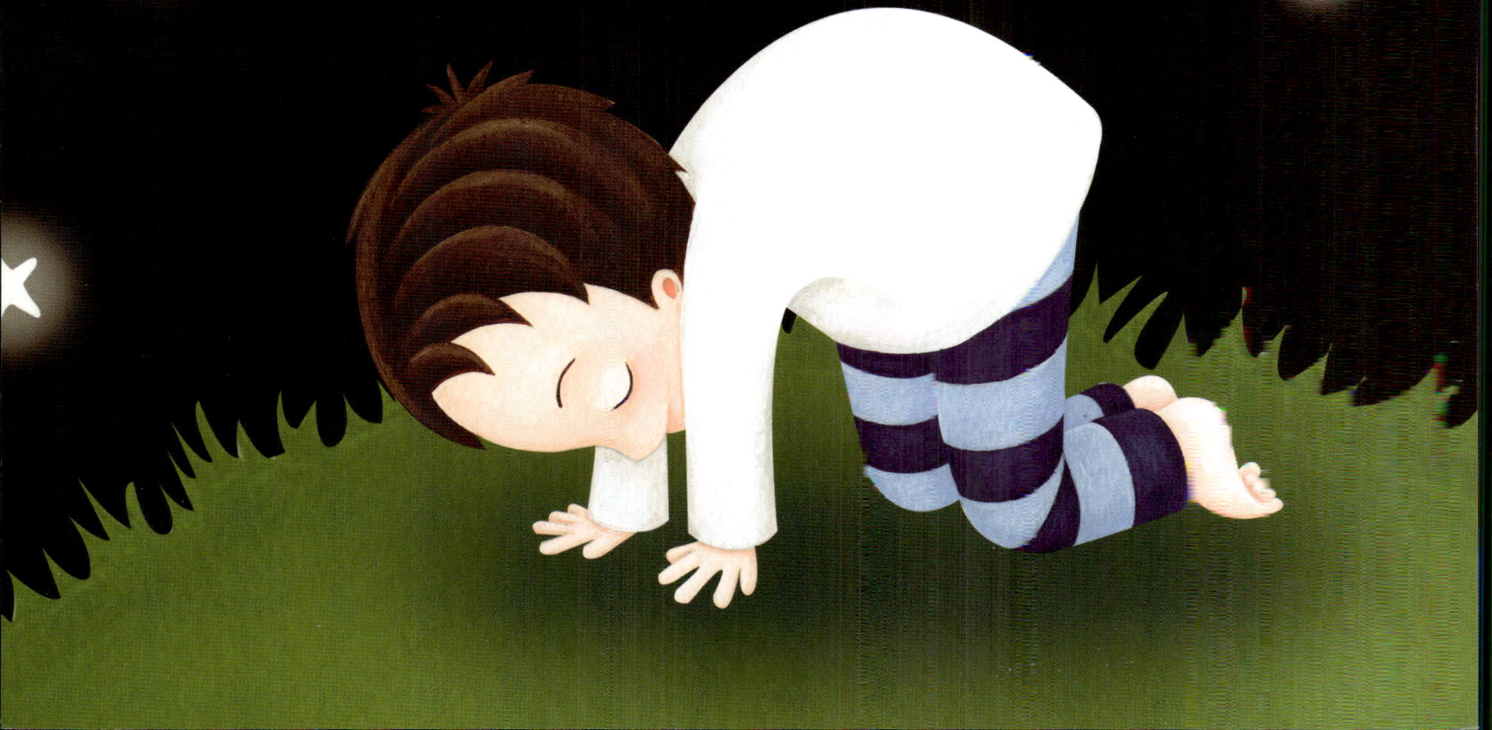

As I breathe in, as I breathe out,
I sit back on my heels,
still and round like the earth.

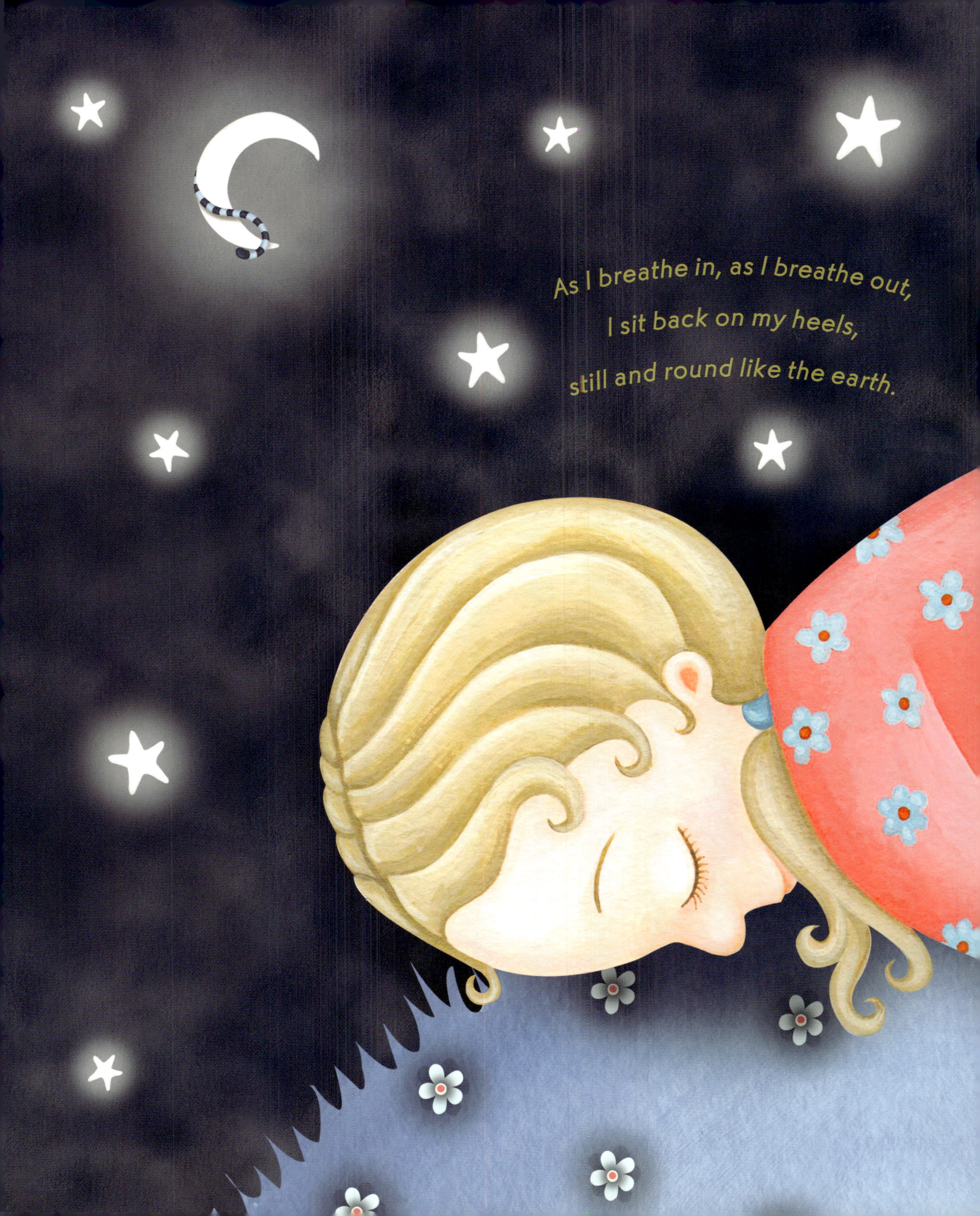

whispers, "Good night world."
You'll be dreaming soon.

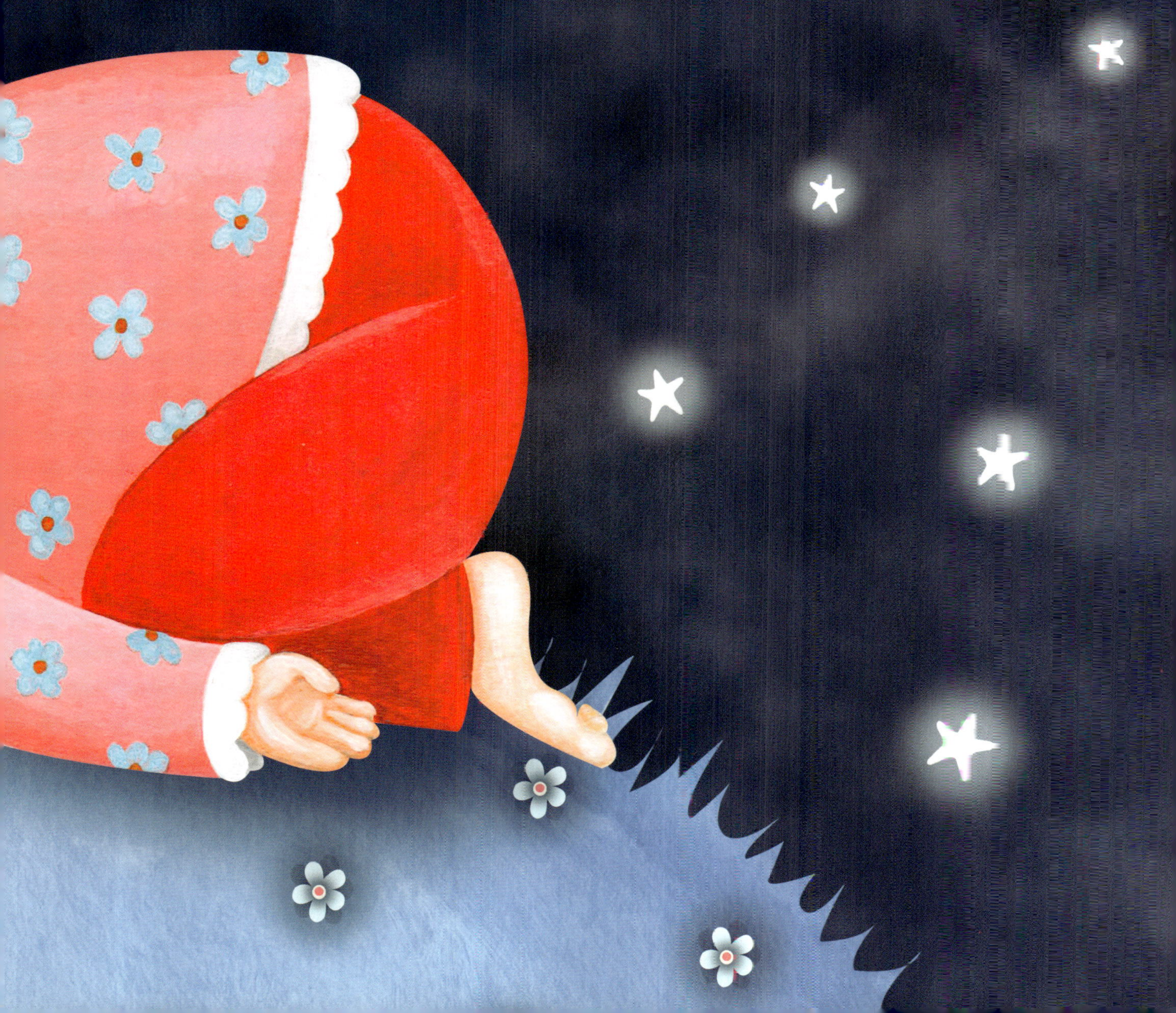

The Good Night Yoga Flow

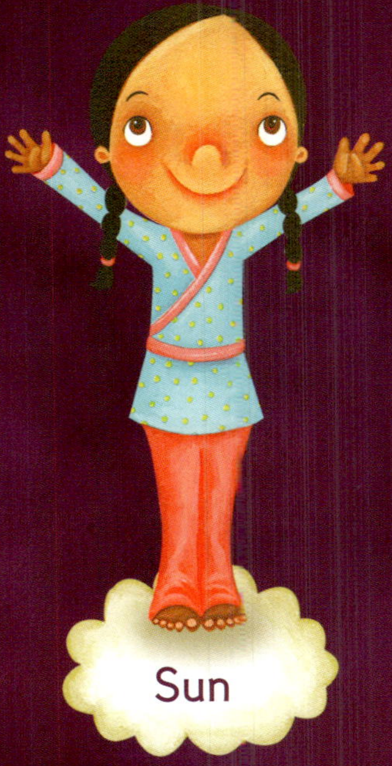

Inhale your arms over your head. Exhale your arms back down.

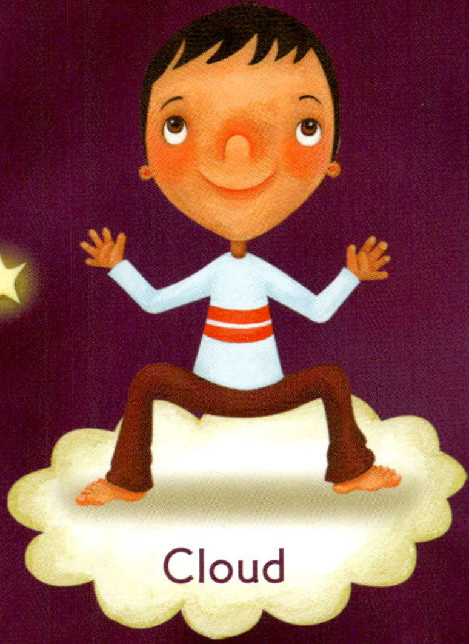

Inhale and bend your knees. Exhale and straighten your legs, lifting your arms above your head.

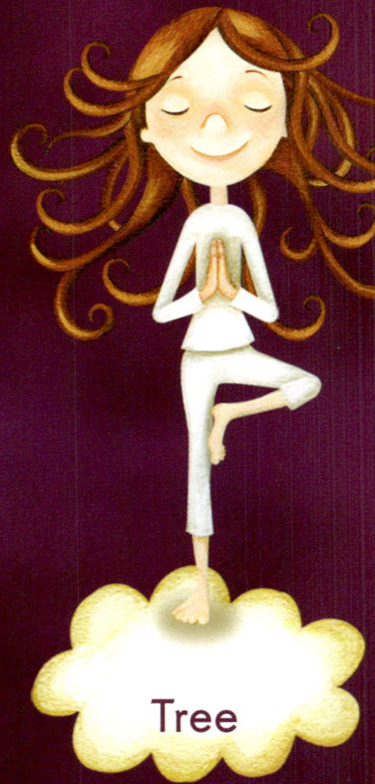

Become tall in your spine. Rest your foot on your ankle or above your knee and balance. Then switch feet.

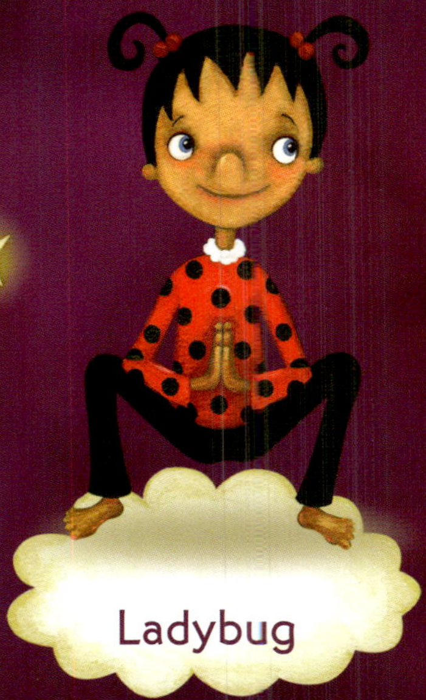

Bend your knees, roll your shoulders back, press your palms together.

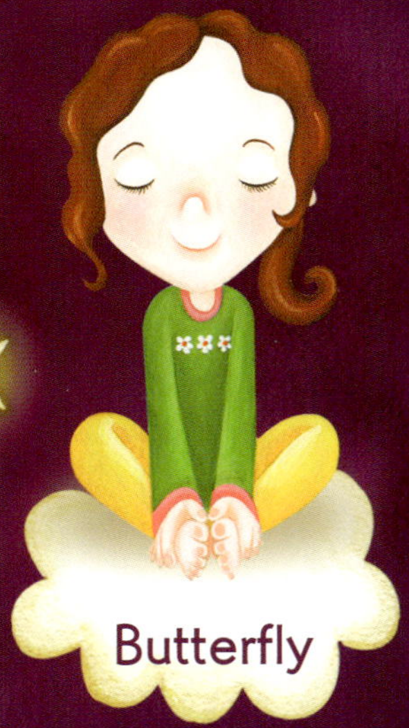

Sit on the ground, press the soles of your feet together, roll your shoulders back.

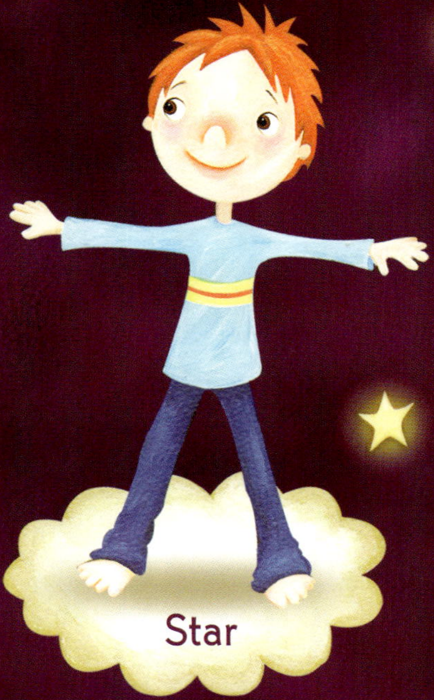

Press down through your feet. Reach your arms out wide.

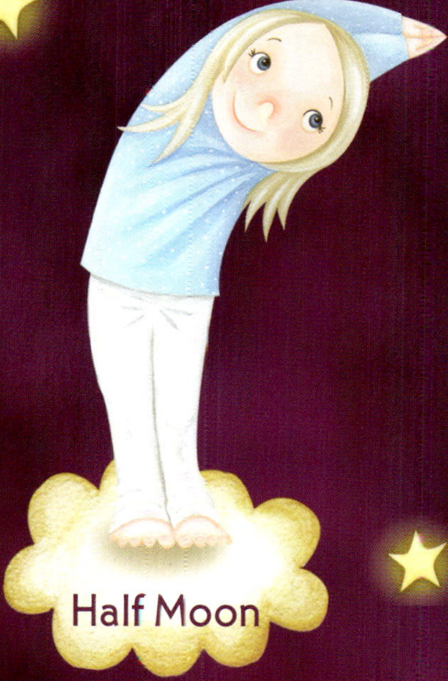

Inhale and lengthen your spine. Exhale and bend to one side, then the other side.

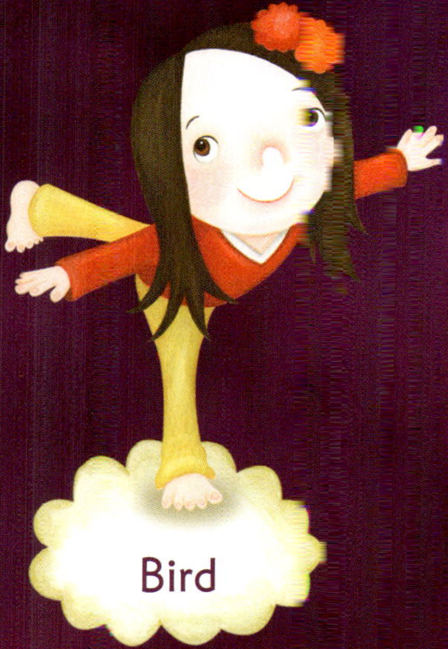

Focus on one point. Lift your foot behind you and balance. Then switch feet.

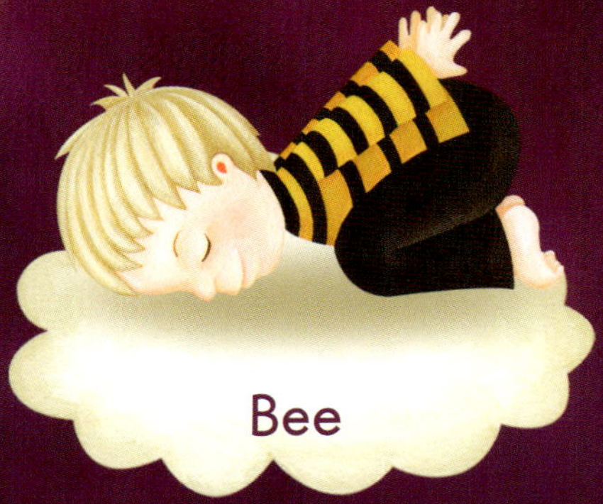

Inhale and sit up straight with your arms back. Exhale and lower your forehead toward the ground.

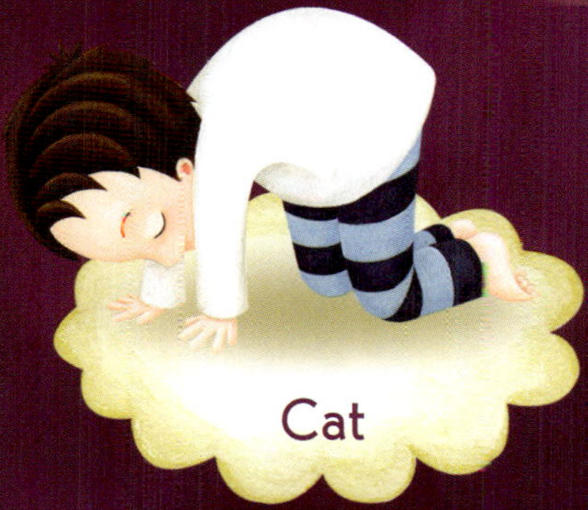

Inhale and look up, letting your spine drop low. Exhale and tuck your chin, lifting your spine high.

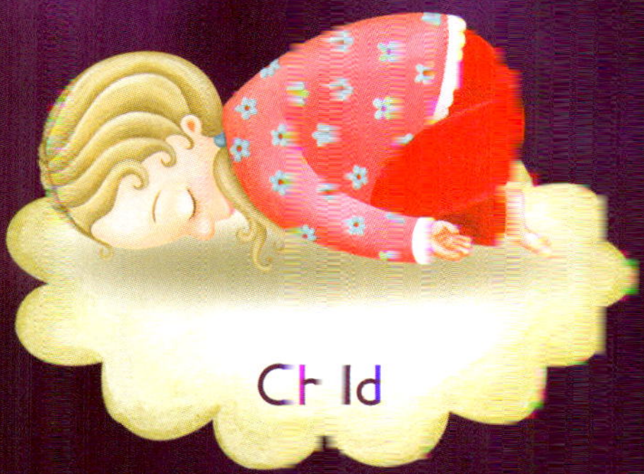

Press back on your heels and rest.

Cloud Journey Visualization

Lie on your back with your hands by your sides.
Take a deep breath in . . . and let a long breath out.
Imagine you are lying on a white, puffy cloud.
Feel yourself sink into its softness as the cloud
lifts you up, up, up into the air.
You are floating. Rocking back . . . and forth.
Your cloud is taking you somewhere you love to be.
This wonderful place has colors to see and sounds to hear.
Feel how good it is to be there.
Breathe in.

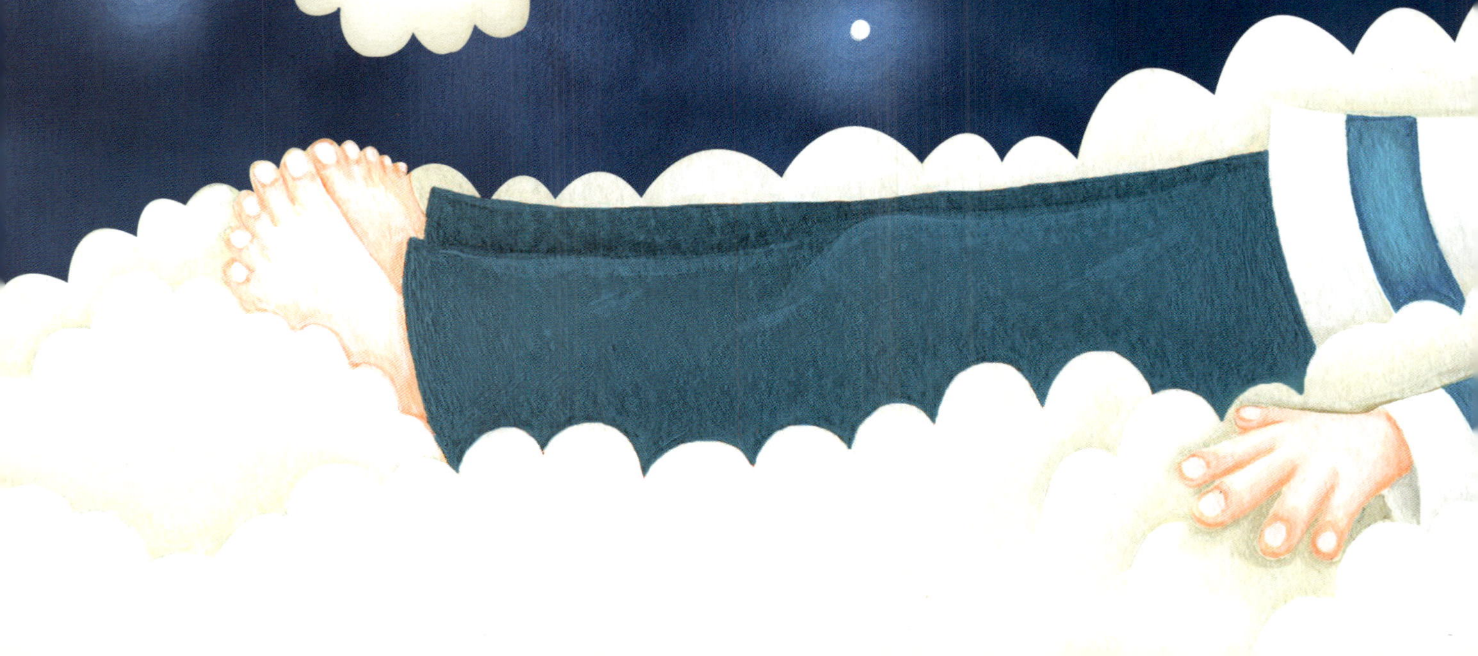

Breathe out.
When you are ready, your cloud
slowly brings you down, down, down.
It settles you gently back on the earth.
As your cloud pulls away, it takes with it anything
that is troubling you—whoosh!
You are left feeling calm, peace,
and happiness inside.
Take another deep breath in . . .
and let a long breath out.
Sweet dreams.

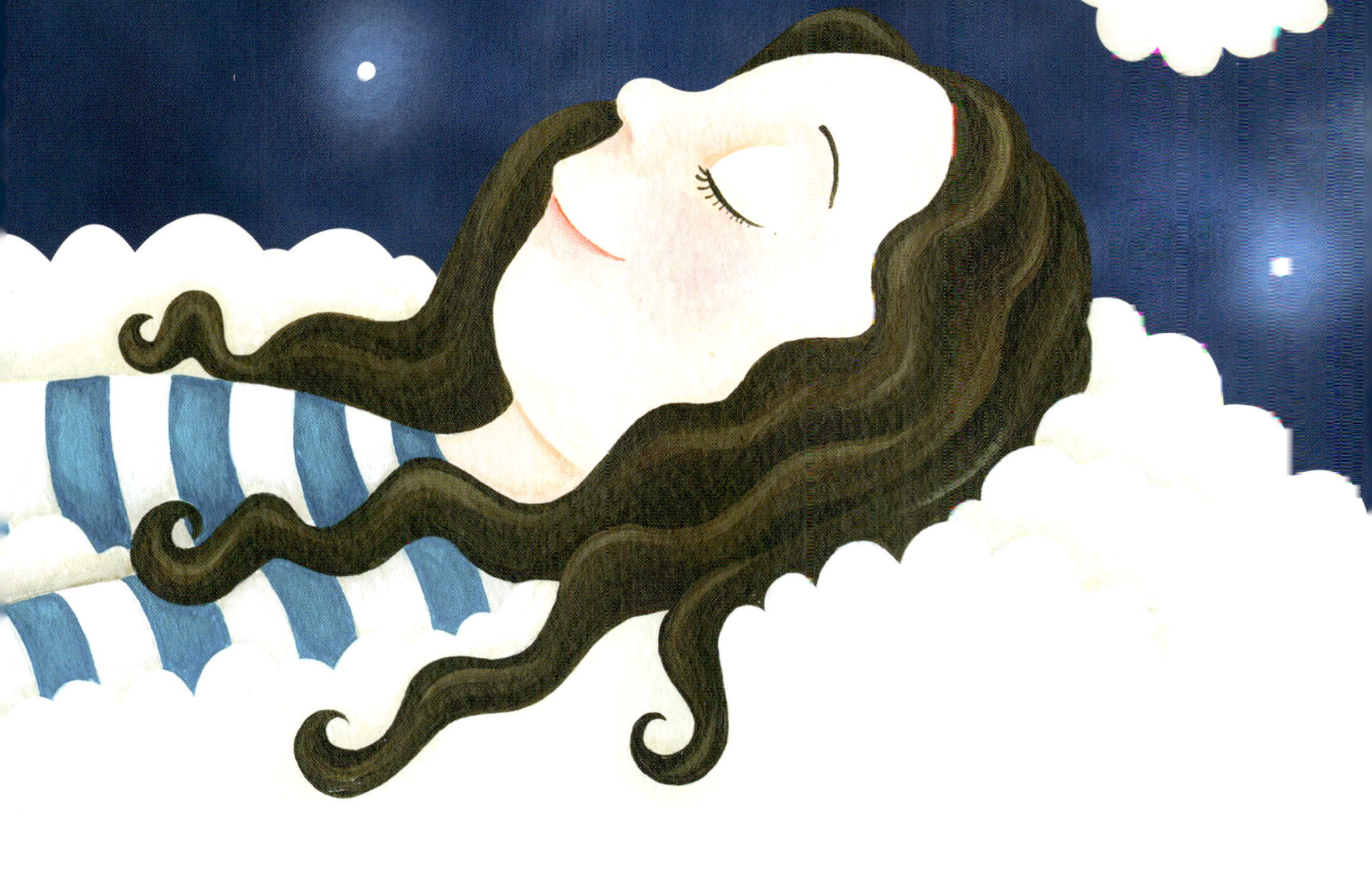

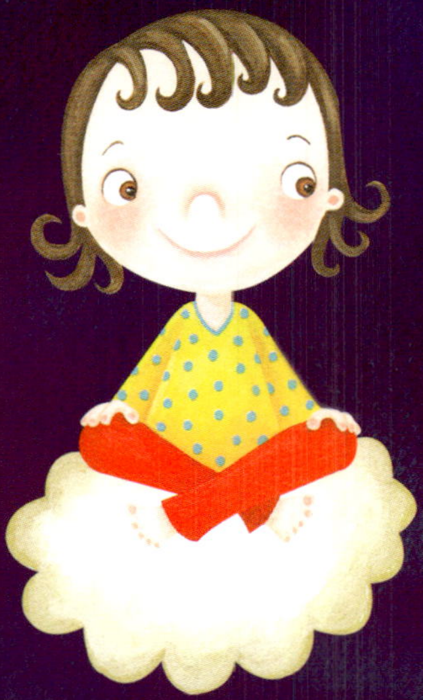

About the Author

As a child, Mariam Gates was a keep-the-light-on, door-open, at-least-one-glass-of-water-by-her-bed sleeper. She has since graduated to "asleep before her head hits the pillow." Mariam holds a master's degree in education from Harvard University and has more than twenty years of experience working with children. Her renowned Kid Power Yoga program combines her love of yoga with teaching to help children access their inner gifts. She lives in Santa Cruz, California, with her husband, yoga teacher Rolf Gates, and their two children. See mariamgates.com.

About the Illustrator

Sarah Jane Hinder discovered her love of illustration as a child when she decided to add some beautiful blue crayon to her nursery-rhyme book—on every single page. As a grownup, she taught art and design for several years before becoming a full-time illustrator. She creates acrylic artwork for a variety of children's books, including *The Three Little Pigs* and *The Elves and the Shoemaker.* She lives in Manchester, England, with her husband and two chihuahuas. See smogawoo.com.

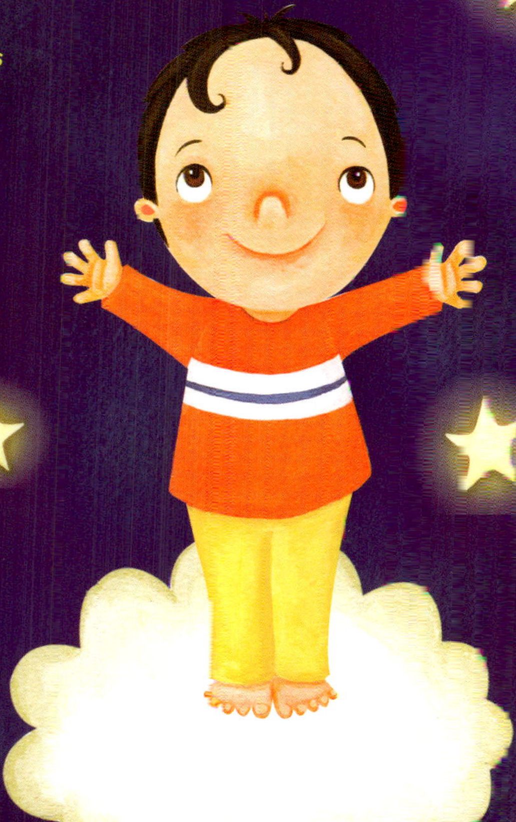

About Sounds True

Sounds True is a multimedia publisher whose mission is to inspire and support personal transformation and spiritual awakening. Founded in 1985 and located in Boulder, Colorado, we work with many of the leading spiritual teachers, thinkers, healers, and visionary artists of our time. We strive with every title to preserve the essential "living wisdom" of the author or artist. It is our goal to create products that not only provide information to a reader or listener, but that also embody the quality of a wisdom transmission.

For those seeking genuine transformation, Sounds True is your trusted partner. At SoundsTrue.com you will find a wealth of free resources to support your journey, including exclusive weekly audio interviews, free downloads, interactive learning tools, and other special savings on all our titles.

To learn more, please visit SoundsTrue.com/freegifts or call us toll-free at 800-333-9185.

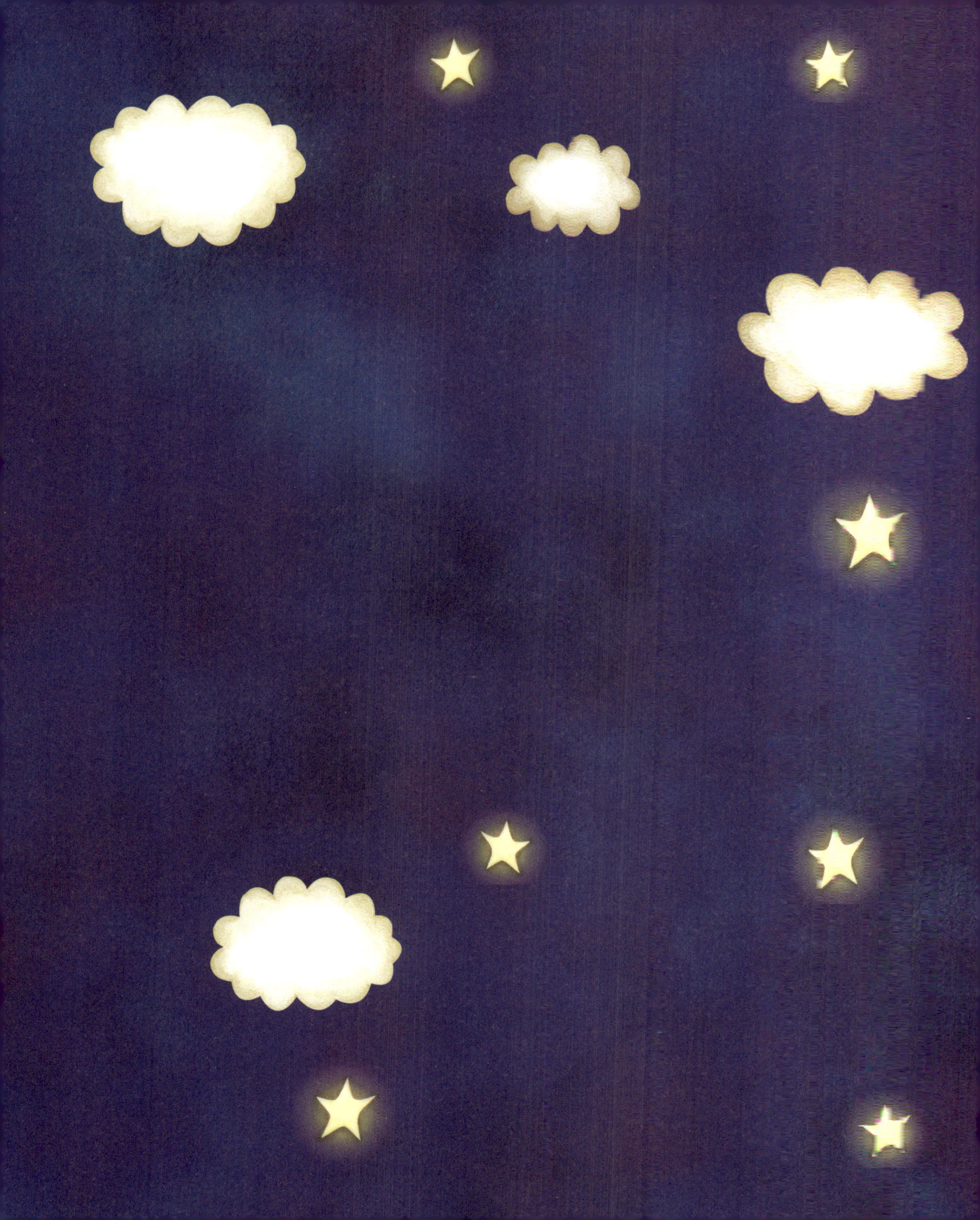

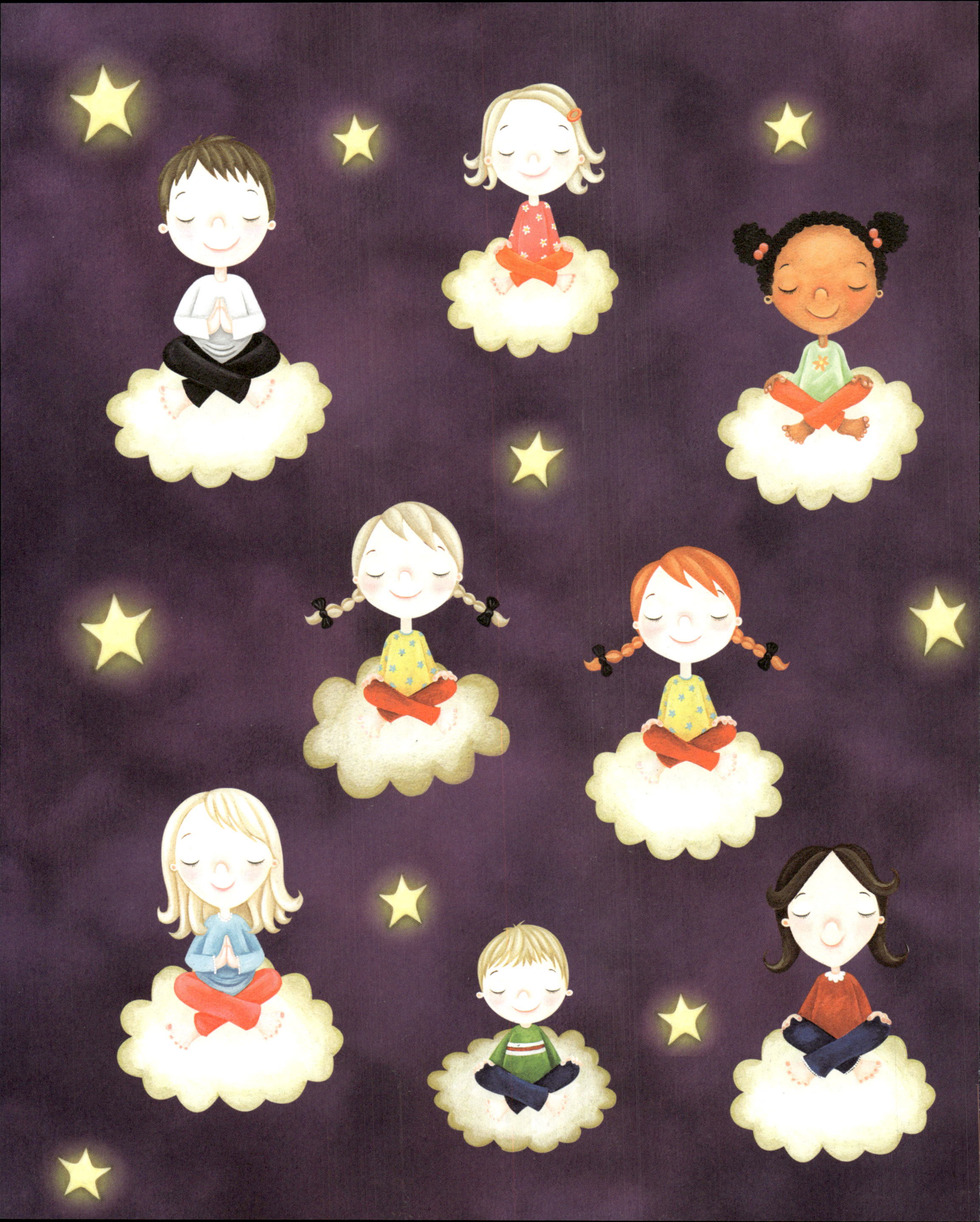